T0251493

Nutrition and Hydration in Hospice Care: Needs, Strategies, Ethics

Nutrition and Hydration in Hospice Care: Needs, Strategies, Ethics

Charlette Gallagher-Allred
Madalon O'Rawe Amenta
Editors

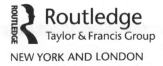

Routledge
Taylor & Francis Group

NEW YORK AND LONDON

First published 1993 by
The Haworth Press, Inc., 10 Alice Street, Binghamton, NY 13904-1580 USA

This edition Published 2014 by Routledge
711 Third Avenue, New York, NY 10017
27 Church Road, Hove, East Sussex, BN3 2FA

Routledge is an imprint of the Taylor & Francis Group, an informa business

Nutrition and Hydration in Hospice Care: Needs, Strategies, Ethics has also been published as *The Hospice Journal,* Volume 9, Numbers 2/3 1993.

© 1993 by The Haworth Press, Inc. All rights reserved. No part of this work may be reproduced or utilized in any form or by any means, electronic or mechanical, including photocopying, microfilm and recording, or by any information storage and retrieval system, without permission in writing from the publisher.

The development, preparation, and publication of this work has been undertaken with great care. However, the publisher, employees, editors, and agents of The Haworth Press and all imprints of The Haworth Press, Inc., including The Haworth Medical Press and Pharmaceutical Products Press, are not responsible for any errors contained herein or for consequences that may ensue from use of materials or information contained in this work. Opinions expressed by the author(s) are not necessarily those of The Haworth Press, Inc.

Library of Congress Cataloging-in-Publication Data

Nutrition and hydration in hospice care : needs, strategies, ethics / Charlette Gallagher-Allred, Madalon O'Rawe Amenta, editors.
    p. cm.
    Has also been published as The Hospice journal, v. 9, no. 2/3, 1993.
    Includes bibliographical references and index.
    ISBN 1-56024-659-6 (alk. paper)
    1. Diet therapy. 2. Terminally ill–Nutrition. 3. Fluid therapy. 4. Hospice care. I. Gallagher-Allred, Charlette R. II. Amenta, Madalon O'Rawe.
    [DNLM: 1. Hospice Care. . Diet. 3. Fluid Therapy. 4. Eating Disorders–therapy. 5. Enteral Nutrition. 6. Parenteral Nutrition. 7. Ethics, Medical. W1 HO69H v. 9, no. 2/3 1993 / WB 310 N976 1993]
RM217.N74 1993
615.8'54–dc20
DNLM/DLC
for Library of Congress
        93-50675
        CIP

ABOUT THE EDITORS

Charlette Gallagher-Allred, RD, PhD, has been a volunteer nutrition consultant at Hospice at Riverside, Columbus, OH since 1979. She is also a nutrition consultant at Ross Laboratories in Columbus, OH, and Clinical Assistant Professor in the Department of Family Medicine at Ohio State University. In addition to *Nutritional Care of the Terminally Ill*, published in 1989 by Aspen Publishers, she is the co-author with John B. Allred of the book *Taking the Fear out of Eating: A Nutritionists' Guide to Sensible Food Choices* published in 1992 by the Cambridge University Press.

Madalon O'Rawe Amenta, RN, DrPH, Vice President of The Hospice Nurses Association and Chairperson of the Professional Advisory Committee of Home Health Services of Allegheny County in Pittsburgh, PA, writes a quarterly column on hospice care for the journal *Home Health Care Nurse* published by J.B. Lippincott. She was Director of Research and Education at the Forbes Hospice in Pittsburgh; founded and served as the first President of the Pennsylvania Hospice Network; and was Mid Atlantic Region Representative to the Board of Directors of the National Hospice Organization. Dr. Amenta has published widely in the hospice care field. She is the first author of the prize-winning book *Nursing Care of the Terminally Ill* published by Little, Brown & Company in 1986 (now available from J.B. Lippincott).

Nutrition and Hydration in Hospice Care: Needs, Strategies, Ethics

CONTENTS

Preface

THE ROLE OF NUTRITION IN HOSPICE CARE

In this volume we address the requirements, strategies, and ethics of nutrition and hydration in hospice care. Nutrition, or food and feeding as we more commonly refer to it, spans the entire course of hospice care and every level of its function from the personal and intimate to the moral and legal.

The Many Meanings of Food and Feeding

At the most fundamental level, food and feeding suggest to us the biological power of sustaining life. Even before the birth of a baby we are mindful of food's special role in producing energy, supporting growth, and maintaining the body. When we are young children food represents the emotional necessities of love, nurturance, appreciation, reward, and belonging. As we grow we come to understand the broader significance of food. We associate it with social and cultural events. We come to expect certain foods on certain occasions–birthdays, holidays, weddings. The offering and sharing of food and drink universally define hospitality. Conversely, the withholding of food is universally regarded on a continuum spanning social slight to cruel and unusual punishment. We understand food symbolically in religious and ethnic terms–body, blood, bread of afflication, dietary laws, fasting, old country or down home cooking, soul food.

[Haworth co-indexing entry note]: "Preface." Gallagher-Allred, Charlette and Madalon O'Rawe Amenta. Co-published simultaneously in *The Hospice Journal* (The Haworth Press, Inc.) Vol. 9, Nos. 2/3, 1993, pp. xvii-xxii: and: *Nutrition and Hydration in Hospice Care: Needs, Strategies, Ethics* (eds: Gallagher-Allred, Charlette, and Madalon O'Rawe Amenta) The Haworth Press, Inc., 1993, pp. ix-xiv. Multiple copies of this article/chapter may be purchased from The Haworth Document Delivery Center [1-800-3-HAWORTH; 9:00 a.m. - 5:00 p.m. (EST)].

© 1993 by The Haworth Press, Inc. All rights reserved.

Food and feeding are a central element and an organizing principle in family life. As noted above, we are concerned with a mother's nutrition during pregnancy both for the health of the child as well as for her own. Through parents, the first purveyors of both food and deep affection, feeding becomes fused in our minds with nurturant behavior. Habits of feeding and eating become distinctive, highly personal, and intimate.

When a family member becomes sick the issue of feeding and eating, then, takes on great significance. Parents want to feed their young children who in turn want to feed their parents when they are aged, mates want to nourish each other, and when the sick and dying person cannot or will not eat it is invariably interpreted as a powerful sign that can mean many things: The biological basis of nutrition is no longer sustaining life, therefore the life is ebbing; the family is losing an essential person in its social system and mealtime is a daily reminder; the caretaker who prepared the food and urged the feeding is losing the role of nurturer; the caretaker who enjoyed the preparation of food as a creative avocation is losing a job. All of these issues can become concerns to the dying patient as well as to the family.

Everyone's heightened awareness resulting from the compression of time for the dying person can raise clinical nutritional problems related to quality of life. Families and patients often need help in the preparation of special foods and ways of adapting to the dying process that can still supply the pleasure, nurturance, and sense of personal control that food and feeding have had for the family and the patient. Many families will think that a nutritional problem—or eating habits or behavior—is the reason the patient became ill. These families will need reassurance to assuage their guilt. Often feeding is the one thing the caretaker can comprehend as a caring and helpful action that she or he can still control and manage alone. As Catherine Maurer Baack notes, "The range of human emotion can be played out over the ingestion of one glass of a dietary supplement."

Ethical and Legal Implications

At the end of the span of hospice care food and feeding are at the core of the biomedical, ethical, and legal problems that have become major controversies in decisions about life-sustaining treatments in our society. The issues of withholding or withdrawing enteral and parenteral nutrition in moribund patients have fueled extensive biomedical ethical debates and generated litigation and in some instances judicial decisions that have been challenged all the way to the Supreme Court.

Nutrition in Hospice Care

Understanding the concerns of patients and their families about nutrition and hydration is essential if hospice care providers are to be successful in helping people live as fully as possible while dealing with death and dying. To address the concerns of patients and their families about nutrition and hydration, we as hospice care providers must explore and become comfortable with our own mortality and the understanding of why we eat and drink as we do. Without such exploration we can have little to say to patients who are forced to confront both their own death and their reasons for accepting or rejecting food and fluid.

The Role of the Dietitian

Because nutrition issues for dying patients and their families are myriad, it is necessary to have a health care professional who understands these issues, who intervenes when appropriate, and who advocates for the patient's and family's wishes. No one is better qualified to interpret and coordinate these concerns than the hospice dietitian. The registered dietitian (RD) performs an essential role in patient and family evaluation, in family and team counseling, and in decision making concerning the moral, ethical, and legal issues surrounding nutrition support for the dying patient.

It is the RD who is most uniquely qualified through education and experience to supervise the assessment and development of the nutrition care plan and to render counseling services in both basic and more complex situations. The RD is the translator of the science of nutrition into the skill of furnishing optimal nourishment to people regardless of state of health. The professionally-trained dietitian also has education in cost control, food safety, and patient acceptance of meals–all critical components of inpatient and day-care hospice programs.

Although basic nutrition assessment and some nutrition counseling is often effectively performed by hospice nursing staff and well-educated volunteers, hospice nurses frequently express a need for more indepth knowledge of the nutritional aspects of care. The RD helps meet this need through providing inservice education programs, individual consultation, and participation in team meetings.

The hospice dietitian should participate in interdisciplinary team meetings, assist the nurse, physician, and volunteers in developing the interdisciplinary plan of care, and serve as a resource on potential nutrient and drug interactions. The RD can also be the administrator's ally by contributing to the development of standards of practice and the policies and procedures that are critical in program operation and accreditation.

One of the most significant dilemmas in hospice care is the timing of the use of artificial nutrition support. Because most hospices do not have policies that either require or bar particular interventions, the RD in conjunction with the nurse and the physician is the appropriate knowledgeable professional to explore the benefits and burdens of artificial nutrition support with the patient, the family, and other team members. The RD and other team members who have built a solid relationship with the patient and family will be able to help the patient and family reach difficult decisions about ethical dilemmas.

Contents of This Volume

The need for nurses to be sensitive to feeding and nutrition issues on a personal level is addressed in the first article, written by an experienced hospice nurse specialist, Catherine Maurer Baack. Only when hospice providers are sensitive to personal feeding and nutrition issues can they form effective partnerships with patients and families that will guide each individual through the storm of emotions and questions that define feeding and nutrition issues.

Practical ways are suggested in several articles in this volume on how to feed and hydrate patients who want to eat, and how to provide support in ways other than feeding for patients who are unable to eat. Constance Holden discusses the troublesome conditions of anorexia, cachexia, and dehydration suggesting appropriate interventions and education for patients and their families. More in-depth information, from the perspective of dietitians Julie O'Sullivan Maillet and Dorothy King, is presented concerning assessment of the patient's nutritional needs, and the role of the dietitian in caring for terminally ill patients and their families. The very special psychosocial and nutritional needs of terminally ill children, their caregivers, and their siblings is sensitively discussed by a team of hospice professionals: nurse administrator Janice Miller-Thiel, ethicist Jacqueline Glover, and dietitian Evelyn Beliveau from Children's Hospice Services in Washington, D.C.

Recognizing the importance of the interdisciplinary team in providing the many services required by the terminally ill patient and family, Phyllis Grauer, a hospice pharmacist, discusses the appropriate use of medications to stimulate appetite in patients who want to eat and who can be helped to do so. Practical considerations necessary to the provision of quality food service and the maximization of quality of life issues for patients and families in inpatient hospice settings are offered by Kathleen Kidd, Director Nutrition and Food Services at The Washington Home and Hospice of Washington and Mary Pat Lane, Manager, Food and Nutrition Services, Hospice of Northern Virginia.

The potential withholding of food and fluids from patients is one of the most controversial and intensely debated issues in modern medical ethics and law. No volume on nutrition in terminal care would be complete without a discussion of its various perspectives. Therefore, the issue of "to feed or not to feed" is addressed in this volume by a variety of hospice professionals: ethicists, physicians, and dietitians. Mark McCamish and Nancy Crocker discuss ethical issues of artificial hydration and nutrition and provide practical information on how to appropriately, enterally and parenterally, feed those patients for whom nutritional support can enhance quality of care and quality of life. Eugene Boisaubin expands on these ethical issues by discussing two important court cases in the past decade that have dealt with the impact of legal decisions for the hospice care of adults and children. He provides guidelines for hospice personnel who deal with end-of-life issues.

The readers of this volume should derive significant insight into the issues of nutrition and hydration for terminally ill patients. It is the hope of the authors and editors that this material will challenge hospice providers to seek ways in which the problems of dying patients and their families can be made easier, and that food and nutrition issues will be considered as important as other palliative care therapies.

We believe that the topics of food, nutrition, and hydration, seldom addressed unless they interject themselves in practice, deserve fuller treatment. Despite the fact that concern about and discussion of nutrition and hydration problems take up a significant portion of hospice care providers' time, the literature in terminal care is sparse concerning them. Only one text in the United States (Gallagher-Allred, 1989) addresses these issues in-depth. We anticipate, therefore, that this volume will provide recognition and thoughtful consideration of material, heretofore notably lacking, that will assist hospice providers in giving the best care possible to terminally ill patients and their families.

Charlette Gallagher-Allred
Madalon O'Rawe Amenta

REFERENCE

Gallagher-Allred, C. R. 1989. *Nutritional care of the terminally ill.* Rockville, MD: Aspen Publishers, Inc.

Nursing's Role in the Nutritional Care of the Terminally Ill: Weathering the Storm

Catherine M. Maurer Baack

SUMMARY. The role of the nurse in nutritional care of the terminally ill is first, to come to terms with personal, psychological, and moral and ethical issues surrounding nutrition and hydration on an individual level; and second, to enter into a partnership with the patient and family and guide them through the storm of emotions and questions using a framework based on principles of ethics, crisis intervention, and effective communication. The nurse's ability to be present with the patient and family during this time is his/her primary tool as the nurse helps them maintain wellness and equilibrium.

INTRODUCTION

Henderson (1966), writes "The unique function of a nurse is to assist the individual sick or well in the performance of those activities contributing to health, or its recovery (or to a peaceful death) that he would perform unaided if he had the necessary strength, will, or knowledge" (p. 15). How, then, can the nurse fulfill this

Catherine M. Maurer Baack, MS, RN, is Clinical Nurse Specialist at Hospice at Riverside, Columbus, OH.

Address correspondence to: Catherine M. Maurer Baack, Hospice at Riverside, 3595 Olentangy River Road, Columbus, OH 43214.

[Haworth co-indexing entry note]: "Nursing's Role in the Nutritional Care of the Terminally Ill: Weathering the Storm." Baack, Catherine M. Maurer. Co-published simultaneously in *The Hospice Journal* (The Haworth Press, Inc.) Vol. 9, Nos. 2/3, 1993, pp. 1-13; and: *Nutrition and Hydration in Hospice Care: Needs, Strategies, Ethics* (eds: Gallagher-Allred, Charlette, and Madalon O'Rawe Amenta) The Haworth Press, Inc., 1993, pp. 1-13. Multiple copies of this article/chapter may be purchased from The Haworth Document Delivery Center [1-800-3-HAWORTH; 9:00 a.m. - 5:00 p.m. (EST)].

© 1993 by The Haworth Press, Inc. All rights reserved.

1

function in interactions with people struggling with the issues surrounding nutrition in the terminally ill?

The process that a patient and family must pursue to sift through their feelings and beliefs and to strain out what is best for them is dynamic and intensely personal. Decisions will come in all shapes and sizes and change frequently at first. The patient and family will try to make these decisions at a time when they are characteristically least able to solve problems, when they are fatigued, stressed, and in crisis. The key to assisting them in this process lies delicately balanced not only in the nurse's technical knowledge and expertise, but also in the nurse's understanding of the individual's basic drive to maintain wellness and equilibrium in his or her life. Interventions based on the principles of: (a) ethical systems, especially in the context of the dying process; (b) crisis intervention; and (c) effective communication are the tools the nurse uses to assist the patient and family to focus on their strengths as they strive for that equilibrium. The following is a discussion of the principles and processes listed above. It is a discussion of not only the science, but also of the art of nursing. It is about not only what a nurse does, but what he or she becomes part of (Leppanen, 1992) as the nurse attempts to weather the storm with terminally ill patients and those close to them.

ETHICAL AND MORAL EXPLORATION

The definition of the function of a nurse as offered by Henderson (1966), when applied in the context of palliative care and nutritional support, most certainly describes a relationship in which the nurse forms a partnership with the patient and family to help them explore the ethical and moral aspects of the decisions they face. To do this, the nurse must explore these issues independently on a personal and professional level for two reasons: (a) to be able to translate and interpret information for the patient and family; and (b) to be sure that the nurse's own values are not imposed on the patient and family (Otte & Allen, 1987).

Bishop and Scudder (1990) write that "nurses need to study clinical ethics so that they can articulate the moral sense inherent in practice" (p. 115). It is this application of ethics to practice that takes the study of ethics from being a philosophical discussion to a way of interacting meaningfully with a patient and family. Bishop and Scudder describe a collegial relationship between patient and family, nurse, and other health care workers that focuses on the process of decision making. This process is centered on a "common devotion to the well-being of the patient" (p. 121). As a result instead of the nurse alone applying ethical principles to a situation, she or he uses these principles as tools to guide all involved toward a decision that will ensure the well-being of the patient.

Scanlon and Flemming (1989) suggest that the best way a nurse can prepare to use ethical principles in the context of treating the terminally ill is to have a clear understanding of the goals of palliative care. They define these goals as the "alleviation of suffering caused by symptoms and the promotion of comfort" (p. 978). Cassell (1991) in his discussion of palliative care writes, "The first aim is that all diagnostic or therapeutic plans be made in terms of the sick person, not the disease. The second is to maximize the patient's function, not the length of life. The third goal is to minimize the suffering of the patient and the family" (p. 241).

Deeper analysis reveals the close relationship between these goals and the principles of ethics most often applied to the care of the terminally ill. Since these principles are discussed as primary topics in other sections of this volume, this paper will not explore them in detail, but refer to them and note how they impact on the well-being of the patient.

Statement of Practitioner's Responsibility

Fundamental to our discussion are two principles that address the practitioner's responsibility as presented by the Hastings Center (1987). They are:

1. The ethical integrity of health care professionals

> Health care professionals have a clear responsibility to act in accordance with the ethical mandates of their professions and reasonable standards of practice. One of their obligations is to respect the considered choice of patient or the patient's surrogate and to affirm the values of compassion and human dignity . . . (and)

2. Justice or equity

> The health care professional's first obligation is to his or her patient. (p. 19-20)

Nutrition and Hydration in the Dying Process

Crucial to the discussion of how to use ethical principles in trying to determine if a treatment such as nutritional support is harmful or just is an understanding of the dying process. It is widely accepted that access to food and water is a basic human need and right. What is not clear, however, is whether this axiom has the same application in all situations. As more is learned about the physiology of dying, the more there is evidence that some forms of nutritional support may be not only ineffectual, but actually potentially harmful. Gallagher-Allred (1991) establishes that due to the physiologic changes caused by an advancing illness and its treatment (e.g., decreased intestinal absorption, slowed gastric emptying, and treatment side effects) anorexia develops and patients tolerate food poorly.

Billings (1985) describes a phenomenon in cancer patients with adequate nutritional intake whose organs, even those not directly affected by the tumor, metabolize nutrients poorly. There is also evidence that the tumor "can be shown to command excessive amounts of nutrients for its own needs" (p. 61). Billings goes on to note that these patients show high rates of protein breakdown and "when they receive parenteral hyperalimentation, they are relatively inefficient in maintaining or increasing their lean body weight or raising their serum albumin as compared with patients with uncomplicated starvation" (p. 61).

Zerwekh (1983) discusses the negative and positive effects of dehydration in the final stages of an illness. She reports that the electrolyte imbalance that occurs as a result of dehydration can cause diminished consciousness, muscle twitching, nausea, vomiting, and a drying of the oral mucosa. However, she also notes that "reduced fluids and increased electrolytes serve almost as natural anesthesia for the central nervous system . . . As the patient's level of consciousness falls, his perception of suffering also decreases" (p. 48). Zerwekh points out that the decreased fluid volume as the result of dehydration ameliorates urinary incontinence and diarrhea;

decreases the pulmonary distress of excessive secretions; and lessens nausea and vomiting in the case of bowel obstruction.

Ultimately, Zerwekh (1983) states the choice regarding nutrition and hydration lies with the patient and family. If the patient wants to be alert and oriented so that he or she may put things in order, then hydration may be indicated. She advises that decisions be "guided by a clinical analysis of the risks and benefits for the patient . . . (and asks) Are I.V. fluids making the patient's discomfort and suffering last longer? . . . and What symptoms are being relieved because the patient's receiving I.V. fluids" (p. 50)? It might be useful to recall in these situations that "stopping treatment is ethically no different from never starting it" (Cassem, 1985, p. 140-141).

CRISIS INTERVENTION

The study of crisis intervention reveals some of the same principles of intervention as does ethical decision making, and provides the nurse with a framework in which to interact with patients and families undergoing a crisis over nutrition concerns. Gaffney (1978) defines crisis as the "experience of one or more people who have a problem or conflict they cannot immediately solve" (p. 14). He states that its nature depends on: (a) factors such as personal and social preparedness to meet change; (b) the environment the individual finds himself in and the resources available to meet change; and (c) the effect the change has had on the individual's perception of his ability to cope.

Blues and Zerwekh (1984) and McGrory (1978) in their explorations of the crisis of death and dying acknowledge that receiving a terminal diagnosis can undoubtedly cause a crisis situation in a patient and family's lives that can lead to disequilibrium. However, depending on how the patient and family meet this crisis, they can either experience increasing disequilibrium and inability to cope; or they can move through the crisis and develop more sophisticated coping mechanisms and growth.

McGrory (1978) proposed a model for the care of the dying based on the belief that all people strive to maintain a level of wellness and equilibrium in their lives even when confronting a terminal illness. In this "Well Model," McGrory (1978) stresses the importance of

building on the strengths of a patient and family as they remain
"active participants . . . represented by a professional person . . . The
strengths all clients possess . . . should be used for support when their
sense of equilibrium and stability is shaken" (p. 26-27).

Steps in Crisis Intervention

Aguilera (1990), Gaffney (1978), and Hoff (1989) outline the
steps to be taken in crisis intervention. They include: (a) assessing
the situation; (b) thoroughly planning an intervention; and (c) implementing the plan and evaluating the plan for the future. These
steps include the following strategies as listed by Hoff (1989):

- Listen actively and with concern . . .
- Encourage the open expression of feelings . . .
- Help the person gain an understanding of the crisis . . .
- Help the individual gradually accept reality . . .
- Help the person explore new ways of coping . . .
- Link the person to a social network . . .
- Reinforce the newly learned coping devices and follow up res-
  olution of crisis. (p. 131-134).

The Nursing Process and Crisis Intervention

A demonstration of how the above applies to nursing is provided
by McGrory (1978) when she superimposes the nursing process
over the steps and strategies of crisis intervention. She writes:

> The first step, assessment, attempts to define the problem and
> elicit coping mechanisms and other valuable resources. The
> second and third steps, planning and intervention, set forth and
> execute care necessary to return the client to the state of equi-
> librium . . . The final step is evaluation and anticipatory plan-
> ning. How well has the situation been resolved? How can what
> the client has learned from this situation help in subsequent
> threatening situations? (p. 82-83)

COMMUNICATION

There is substantial agreement among several authors (Aguilera,
1990; Blues & Zerwekh, 1989; Gaffney, 1978; McGrory, 1978) that

effective intervention hinges on communicating well enough with the patient and family to, at least, assist them back to a precrisis level of function, and at most to "allow new coping patterns to emerge that can help the individual function at a higher level of equilibrium than before the crisis" (Aguilera, 1990, p. 70-71). Communication is more than the presentation of accurate information. It is also the building of relationships and rapport (Hoff, 1989). Communication is listening, sharing ideas, and at times, touch (Reardon & Beckmann, 1979; McGrory, 1978). Jametown (1984) states that "mystery and dread can be staved off by acts as simple as holding hands" (p. 226).

Guidelines for Communication

General guidelines for communication include (Reardon & Beckmann, 1979; Hoff, 1989; McGrory, 1978):

- Being aware of the psychological, social, and cultural makeup of all persons involved, including that of health care professional;
- Being sure to convey an open, honest, and caring attitude in each situation;
- Allowing the patient and family to set the pace of the conversation;
- Using open-ended questions and reflective statements to encourage verbalization and clarification of issues;
- Avoiding professional jargon;
- Validating each individual's feelings to insure that he or she feels heard;
- Learning to be comfortable with silences and to trust that being is as important as talking.

Being Present During Professional Communication

Being present with someone during stressful times is often what that person will remember the most. Words often fail during stressful moments. McGrory (1978) writes that "talking with the dying is filled with land mines" (p. 126). And Hoff (1989) writes:

The most technically flawless communication skills are useless in absence of rapport with a person in crisis. Conversely, if
our values, attitudes, and feelings about a person are re-
spectful, unprejudiced, and based on true concern, those
values will almost always be conveyed to the person regardless of possible technical errors in communication. (p. 116)

Case Example

The discussion above takes on more meaning when examined in
the light of a struggle of a young woman who called a hospice
program one afternoon asking to talk to someone–anyone who
could help her. She explained she knew very little about hospice,
only that hospice helped people who were dying and her father was
dying. He was in an intensive care unit on a ventilator, receiving
total parenteral nutrition, and totally unresponsive. She knew he
would never leave the hospital, and in that respect admitted feeling
foolish calling an agency she knew she would never use. She was
desperate.

Her father was dying from emphysema. That morning, his physician told her that he felt her father would never be able to be weaned
off the ventilator and would continue to decline–most probably
never to regain consciousness. The physician talked with the
woman about taking her father off all artificial life support. Her
question to the hospice staff member–"What do I do?"

This woman was struggling for equilibrium. Her father had been
seriously ill and on life support several times before. She was accustomed to the routine. The knowledge that this time was different put
her in the position of facing her father's death as a whole new
reality. His death was no longer somewhere in the future–it was
here and now, and she believed she was being asked to cause it to
happen.

Following the strategies of crisis intervention outlined above, the
nurse counseling this young woman listened to her unfolding story
and offered acknowledgement and validation for the woman's feelings and concerns. The nurse, in time, gradually started to explore
this woman's ethical concerns about causing her father's death in
light of the biomedical ethical and moral principles.

The nurse invited the young woman to incorporate these ideas in her decision making and encouraged her to trust her own ability to make a good decision. The nurse gave her name to the woman and asked her permission to talk with her father's physician as well, so as to keep an avenue open for further discussion and support if needed. A summary of the content of the nurse's intervention follows:

> It sounds like you are really struggling with this decision. If you feel you are being asked to make a life or death decision, it may be helpful to look at your problem from a different perspective. Your father has terminal emphysema. He cannot be cured. In a way the decision about his living and dying has already been made. His crisis this time is not just another setback. You know he will die sooner or later in spite of the life support measures.

> The decision you are asked to make now is one about the quality of your father's life. Would he want this (being on life support) for himself? Only you can answer this in your heart of hearts from what you have learned about your father throughout your life. There is no right or wrong answer, just the answer you find within yourself. Please call back if you need to talk again. With your permission I would like to speak to your father's physician to let him know that you have spoken with me and to offer my continuing support.

THE ROLE OF THE NURSE

Throughout interactions with the terminally ill patient and his or her loved ones, the nurse draws from resources that can only be framed within the art of nursing. The nurse must assist the family in repairing the fabric of their lives now torn apart by the storm of a terminal diagnosis. Just as the weaver must have all the materials for his loom—warp, weft, and shuttle to join form and color—so too the patient and family need the necessary technical information, the ethical and moral subtleties, and the coping mechanisms to rejoin the fabric of their lives.

Bishop and Scudder (1990) write that "although legally the patient has the right to make decisions about what is good for him, morally, that decision should be made by the physician, nurse, and patient working together" (p. 136). Each person brings to the interaction information, knowledge, and expertise that, when woven together, reveals what is going to provide optimal well-being for the patient and family. This interaction between patient, family, and health care professional is the essence of good health care.

The nurse's part in this interaction is one in which she or he must be able to make peace with ambiguity and become part of the process. The terms advocate, mediator, and facilitator all come to the fore as the nurse begins to listen, to educate, to redefine, and reframe information in order to revitalize the patient's and family's coping mechanisms. This approach is not comfortable nor does it come easily. It is easy to have an opinion. It is not easy to just be.

Case Examples

For the nurse interacting with a man faced with the decision of withholding hydration and nutrition from his dying wife who says, "I was a prisoner of war. I know what it is like to be hungry and thirsty, and she will not go through that," it is essential to listen to his description of his own pain as well as to hear his need to protect and defend his wife of over 50 years. It is important to validate his beliefs as legitimate and yet invite him to reframe his beliefs in a way that more closely reflects the reality of his wife's condition. He needs to be encouraged to verify his beliefs with his wife and physician, and then he needs to be offered other ways of showing how much he cares for her. The nurse might respond:

> Mr. G., I hear what your are saying to me about your experience as a prisoner of war. Malnutrition and dehydration in a healthy person is indeed painful and very harmful. However, Mr. G., your wife is very ill and her body is weak. To artificially provide food and hydration may place an undue burden on her body which is already burdened enough with trying to compensate for what the tumor is doing to it.
>
> I think it may be a good idea to ask your wife if she is feeling hungry and thirsty and how much it is bothering her. I en-

courage you to talk it over with her and your doctor as to whether your wife wants the I.V. It is obvious that you love your wife very much and we can help you find several ways to make sure your wife is comfortable.

Gallagher-Allred (1989) calls this type of interaction an attempt "to diminish the no-win situation. Teaching the family about the effects that the disease and dying have on eating is important. The family's anxieties can be diminished and the patient can be freed from the pressure to eat when you help the family shift attention from maintaining the patient's nutritional status to enhancing patient comfort through providing small appetizing meals . . . Although this shift may be difficult at first for the family, it brings considerable relief to both patient and family in the long run" (Gallagher-Allred, 1989, p. 220).

This approach was also used by a nurse to interact with a frantic woman who said of her dying husband, "I just can't watch him starve."

> The fact that your husband is not eating does not mean starvation in the same way that people starve in a famine. His loss of appetite is the result of his body shutting down and it is a natural part of the dying process. You are not letting him down or neglecting him. In fact, by giving him small amounts of his favorite foods when he asks for them, you are going to make him more comfortable.

A final example. A woman with a 1.5 cm pressure sore that would not heal cried because it wouldn't improve but she couldn't force herself to eat the nutrients that would help. It became apparent that she was focusing on the sore to the exclusion of everything else in her life. She appeared to be caught in a downward spiral of emotions and recriminations. A change in focus appeared to be what might be needed. The nurse's intervention went as follows:

> This bed sore really worries you. What bothers you the most about this sore? (The patient started to cry) 'I'm not going to get better. I'm going to die.'

The woman had transferred all her fears about dying and hopes for living to the healing of a tiny pressure sore. When it became possible for her to speak directly about her hopes and fears, the concern over the pressure sore diminished.

Of course, the above interactions were highly condensed for the purposes of this paper. Most took place over several home visits. The purpose in recounting them is to share some insights that have proved helpful and to underscore the importance of trusting one's ability to be present with people. Bishop and Scudder (1990) write, "Dilemmas by their nature cannot be solved; they simply must be faced. However, they need not be faced alone" (p. 122).

CONCLUDING THOUGHTS

It is imperative that the nurse take the time to pursue the decision making process personally. In this way, when confronted with these issues in the context of assisting a patient and family, the nurse can provide the support needed as the patient and family strive to make their decisions. The most important tool any nurse will ever have as he or she weathers the storm of a terminal illness with a patient and family is the tool named–Self.

REFERENCES

Aguilera, D. C. (1990). *Crisis intervention: Theory and methodology*. St. Louis: C.V. Mosby.

Billings, J. A. (1985). *Outpatient management of advanced cancer: Symptom control, support, and hospice-in-the-home*. Philadelphia: J. B. Lippincott.

Bishop, A. H., & Scudder, J. R., Jr. (1990). *The practical, moral, and personal sense of nursing: A phenomenological philosophy of practice*. New York: State University of New York Press.

Blues, A. G., & Zerwekh, J. V. (1984). *Hospice and palliative nursing care*. Orlando, FL: Grune and Stratton.

Cassell, E. J. (1991). *The nature of suffering: And the goals of Medicine*. New York: Oxford University Press.

Cassem, E. H. (1985). Appropriate treatment limits in advanced cancer. In J. M. Billings (Ed.), *Outpatient management of advanced cancer: Symptom control, support, and hospice-in-the-home* (pp. 139-151). Philadelphia: J.B. Lippincott.

Gaffney, T. (1978). Crisis intervention–basic theory and methodology. In Wicks, R. J., Fine, J. A., & Platt, J. J. (Eds.), *Crisis intervention: A practical, clinical guide* (pp. 7-23). USA: Charles B. Slack.

Gallagher-Allred, C. R. (1989). *Nutritional care of the terminally ill.* Rockville, MD: Aspen.

Gallagher-Allred, C. R. (1991). Nutritional care of the terminally ill patient and family. In Penson, J., & Fisher, R. (Eds.), *Palliative care for people with cancer.* (pp. 91-104). London, England: Hodder & Stoughton.

Hastings Center. (1987). *Guidelines on the termination of life-sustaining treatment and the care of the dying.* Briarcliff Manor, NY: The Hastings Center.

Henderson, V. (1966). *The nature of nursing.* New York: Harper.

Holden, C. M. (1991). Anorexia in the terminally ill cancer patient: The emotional impact on the patient and the family. *The Hospice Journal, 7*(3), 73-84.

Hoff, L. A. (1989). *People in crisis: Understanding and helping* (3rd ed.). Redwood City, CA: Addison-Wesley.

Jametown, A. (1984). *Nursing practice: The ethical issues.* Englewood Cliffs, NJ: Prentice Hall.

Leppanen, M. C. (1992). Caring vs. curing. *Hospice, 3*(3), 20-23.

McGrory, A. (1978). *A well model approach to the care of the dying client.* New York: McGraw-Hill.

Otte, D. M., & Allen, K. S. (1987). Ethical principles in the nursing care of the terminally ill adult. *Cancer Nursing Perspectives, 14*(5), 87-91.

Reardon, C. M., & Beckmann, M. R. (1979). *Dying in an institution.* New York: Appleton-Century-Crofts.

Scanlon, C., & Fleming, C. (1989). Ethical issues in caring for the patient with advanced cancer. *Nursing Clinics of North America, 24*(4), 977-984.

Zerwekh, J. V. (1983, January). The dehydration question. *Nursing, 83,* 47-51.

Nutrition and Hydration in the Terminally Ill Cancer Patient: The Nurse's Role in Helping Patients and Families Cope

Constance M. Holden

SUMMARY. Cancer patients and their family members must cope with multiple losses as the disease progresses. The loss of ability to eat and drink is a real and perceived harbinger of the ultimate loss: death. While health care professionals know that these physiologic changes are a normal part of the dying process, families are rarely able to accept them easily. Because these losses have such profound emotional, spiritual, and physical ramifications, it is important that staff be prepared to provide appropriate support and information to patients and families. The suggestions posed in this article may be utilized by all members of the interdisciplinary team.

INTRODUCTION

Anorexia and cachexia are among the most frequently reported symptoms of advanced cancer (Wachetal, Allen-Masterson, Reu-

Constance M. Holden, RN, MSN, is Manager of North Hospice at North Memorial Medical Center in Robbinsdale, MN.

Adddress correspondence to: Constance M. Holden, North Hospice, North Memorial Medical Center, 3300 Oakdale North, Robbinsdale, MN 55422.

[Haworth co-indexing entry note]: "Nutrition and Hydration in the Terminally Ill Cancer Patient: The Nurse's Role in Helping Patients and Families Cope." Holden, Constance M. Co-published simultaneously in *The Hospice Journal* (The Haworth Press, Inc.) Vol. 9, Nos. 2/3, 1993, pp. 15-35: and: *Nutrition and Hydration in Hospice Care: Needs, Strategies, Ethics* (eds: Gallagher-Allred, Charlette, and Madalon O'Rawe Amenta) The Haworth Press, Inc., 1993, pp. 15-35. Multiple copies of this article/chapter may be purchased from The Haworth Document Delivery Center [1-800-3-HAWORTH; 9:00 a.m. - 5:00 p.m. (EST)].

© 1993 by The Haworth Press, Inc. All rights reserved.

15

ben, Goldberg, & Mor, 1988). A 1985 survey of the staff of 100 hospice programs across the country revealed that anorexia, experienced by 60% of their patients, was the most frequently reported nutritional problem (Simonetti, 1985). Patients and especially their caregivers respond to the patient's loss of ability to eat with the same emotions that accompany any loss: anger, fear, frustration, sadness, and less often–acceptance (Holden, 1991). Amenta and Bohnet (1986) suggest that the family that associates food with love will have a particularly difficult time coping with the anorectic patient. Families, who rarely know that the inability to eat and to drink is a normal part the disease progression and the dying process, often harbor the expectation that medical interventions will ameliorate these symptoms. It may be extremely difficult for family members to cope with such an emotion-laden loss.

In a study comparing patient and family member perception of the patient's anorexia, it was noted that while family members rated anorexia as a major concern, the patients, themselves, were likely to be more concerned about other symptoms (Holden, 1991). All members of the hospice team will be aware of the patient's and the family's struggle to cope with this problem. While there are no clear lines of role demarcation, this discussion will focus on the nurse's responsibilities, which include:

- Assessing each patient/family situation,
- Suggesting appropriate interventions,
- Providing education for patients/families and others,
- Helping families cope with the emotional aspects of this loss.

Although the emotional responses to the lost ability to eat and to drink are similar, for purposes of clarity, this discussion will be divided into two segments: (1) anorexia, cachexia, and malnutrition; and (2) dehydration in the imminently dying patient.

ANOREXIA, CACHEXIA, AND MALNUTRITION

Researchers at the Cross Cancer Institute in Edmonton, Alberta, found significant malnutrition present in 51% of patients with advanced cancer and in 80% of those in the terminal state (Bruera &

MacDonald, 1988). They classified the causes of malnutrition into three categories: (1) decreased intake, (2) increased caloric needs related to the malignancy, and (3) malabsorption.

Decreased Intake

Food intake can be impaired by a number of factors, but significant problems are caused by abnormalities in taste sensation and by nausea and vomiting. These symptoms may be caused by the disease or the treatment. Bernstein (1986) contends that, in addition to tumor-induced food aversions, it is likely that the patient will develop learned aversions to food that are commonly associated with chemotherapy or tumor growth.

Poorly managed symptoms such as nausea, vomiting, pain, dyspnea, or constipation can contribute greatly to the patient's inability to eat. Unfortunately, the medications employed in the treatment of the disease and in the control of symptoms may also negatively affect appetite. Constipation, a common side effect of narcotic administration, unless conscientiously managed, may lead to an impaction and/or to nausea and vomiting. Narcotics may also cause dry mouth (xerostomia) and nausea and vomiting. Other contributors to a significant degree of xerostomia include phenothiazines, diuretics, and tricyclic antidepressants. Non-steroidal anti-inflammatory drugs (NSAIDs) may also induce a level of gastro-intestinal distress that impairs food intake. The physician and the nurse must collaborate regularly, assessing the cause and effect relationship between the symptoms being managed and the side effects that affect a patient's appetite.

Cachexia and Malnutrition

Cachexia, profound and progressive bodily wasting, and weight loss are significant problems for end-state cancer patients. Ohnuma (1989) among others has noted that the interrelated syndromes of anorexia, cachexia, and malnutrition are major causes of morbidity in patients with advanced disease. As early as 1932, Warren proposed malnutrition as a major cause of cancer deaths.

The Role of Total Parenteral Nutrition (TPN)

Despite the negative impact of malnutrition on survival, aggressive nutritional support, consisting of total parenteral nutrition (TPN) or enteral feedings, has not been successful in reversing the above-mentioned symptoms in most patients. Patients who do benefit, however, include those who have intestinal obstructions but who have not already lost body weight, those whose treatment regimens are expected to be effective, patients suffering radiation-induced enteritis, and children with lymphoma and leukemia (Ohnuma, 1989).

Conversely, and worthy of concern, there are studies indicating that patients being treated with TPN may have a shortened survival time because the enhanced nutrition may enhance tumor growth (Shika & Brennan, 1989; Torosian & Daly, 1986). Other studies indicate that artificially administered sustenance has no significant impact on tumor response to radiation or chemotherapy (Bruera & MacDonald, 1988). Even when TPN has achieved weight maintenance, it has been through water and fat accumulation rather than improved protein status (Souba & Copeland, 1989). Kaye (1990) and Bruera and MacDonald (1988) assert emphatically that neither enteral or parenteral feedings have a place in the clinical management of patients with advanced cancer.

It is important that the hospice nurse have knowledge of these findings. Reference may be made to them when educating patients, family members, staff, and volunteers who may be suggesting that these interventions be employed.

NURSING ASSESSMENT OF THE NUTRITIONAL ASPECTS OF THE PATIENT AND THE FAMILY

As indicated above, terminally ill patients have significant problems with nutrition upon admission to a hospice program. The first component in providing appropriate nutritional care is a thorough assessment of the patient and of the family. The initial screening should take place upon admission whenever possible and appropriate. Such a screening will identify areas of concern and the need for consultation by a dietitian. Figure 1 is an example of a screening instrument that could be used by the nurse to conduct a preliminary assessment.

The nurse needs access to information concerning the patient's disease, prognosis, pattern of metastasis, current and past therapies, and prescribed medications and their effectiveness. Information may be obtained from the patient and family about related symptoms such as nausea, vomiting, diarrhea, constipation, mouth sores, and/or dysphagia. The extent of the anorexia may be discerned from a description of the past 24 hours of intake. It is also helpful to know the patient's pre-illness weight as well as her or his present weight.

An assessment should be made of the patient's and the family's emotional responses to the eating difficulties. Initially, it may be useful to have separate discussions with the patient and the family members to elicit the most honest expressions of feelings. There is often a high degree of anger and frustration, especially on the part of the caregiver, who is focused on feeding the patient (Amenta & Bohnet, 1986).

Hospice nurses report that, for the family, the quantity of food and fluid taken serves as a barometer of the patient's well-being. This is often the first information offered when a family is queried about the patient's condition. While other bodily functions may also be deteriorating, it is the patient's intake that is most noticed by the family.

Suggesting Appropriate Interventions

The appropriateness of interventions is determined by the patient's diagnosis, prognosis, and desires. For a patient who has mild appetite loss and mild food aversions, but who wants to and can eat, the suggestions and recipes in *Eating Hints* (National Cancer Institute, 1987), a cookbook produced by the National Cancer Institute, may be useful. Helpful suggestions include serving food and fluids in small amounts, selecting cool and non-odorous foods, avoiding red meats or other foods that commonly cause aversions, and enriching milk products with powdered protein additives. Gallagher-Allred (1989) offers comprehensive treatment suggestions for managing nutrition-related problems. Figure 2 addresses the management of anorexia.

FIGURE 1. Preliminary Nutritional Assessment–Hospice

1. Which of the following are troubling to the patient or the family?
   - Poor intake of food   Yes _____ No _____
   - Inability to eat certain foods   Yes _____ No _____
   - Specify _____
   - Vomiting   Yes _____ No _____
   - Nausea   Yes _____ No _____

   Is the nausea associated with certain foods, the sight or smell of foods, medications, depression or anxiety? Are medications being taken to control the nausea and vomiting and how effective are they?
   - Dry Mouth   Yes _____ No _____
   - Sore Mouth   Yes _____ No _____
   - Difficulty Swallowing   Yes _____ No _____
   - Constipation   Yes _____ No _____

2. Does the patient have the following?
   - Colostomy   Yes _____ No _____
   - Feeding Tube   Yes _____ No _____
   - Intravenous Infusion   Yes _____ No _____
   - Total Parenteral Nutrition   Yes _____ No _____
   - Other   Yes _____ No _____

3. What are the patient's feelings about the changes in eating patterns?

4. What are the family members' feelings about the patient's eating problems? About his/her role change resulting from the patient not eating?

5. What do the patient or family members know about the causes of the patient's eating difficulties?

6. Would the patient or family member like to discuss any concerns with a dietitian?   Yes _____ No _____

Rarely is the practice of conducting a calorie count appropriate because it can be a cruel reminder of the patient's inadequate intake. Neither does monitoring the patient's weight provide useful information. If the patient's disease is advanced and the loss of appetite profound, it is most appropriate to recommend food and fluids only as she or he requests. In truth, most patients would prefer to have their families focus less on eating problems; they would prefer, themselves, to control the amount and nature of food served to them (Holden, 1991).

Services of the Registered Dietitian

The services of a registered dietitian (RD) who is trained in palliative care, may be useful. The RD is qualified through education and experience to supervise the assessment process and to guide the team in the development of a nutritional care plan. She or he may counsel patients and families, provide staff and volunteer education, attend team meetings and serve as a resource to the entire interdisciplinary group (Gallagher-Allred, 1989).

Medical Therapies That Aid Appetite and Intake

For the patient who wants to eat and can be helped to do so, the dietitian and nurse should employ their best counseling skills, and they should also consider the following medical assists:

- Steroids–Dexamethasone 4 mg per day or prednisone 30 mg per day may be effective as an appetite stimulant (Kaye, 1990).
- Hormones–There is some evidence that megestrol acetate (Megace) and medroxyprogesterone may stimulate increased appetite and weight gain in some patients with breast cancer (Bruera & MacDonald, 1988).
- Metoclopramide–If the patient's anorexia seems to be related to delayed gastric emptying, 10 mg of metoclopramide may be effective (Kaye, 1990).
- Antiemetics–A careful assessment of the patient's nausea and vomiting may yield information related to etiology. This will enable the physician to prescribe the most effective antiemetic.
- Total parenteral nutrition or gastrostomy tube feeding.

FIGURE 2. The Management of Anorexia

Symptoms and Cause of Symptoms	Drug Management
Tumor effects: pelvic/abdominal mass, liver metastases, abdominal compression, constipation	Appetite stimulants: prednisone amitriptyline beer or wine or sherry
Treatment effects: postsurgical stasis or small stomach, drug treatment, chemotherapy, radiation therapy, mouth and esophageal pain, dental problems, loss of teeth	Thorazine antidepressants Periactin Megace
Taste changes: early satiety, unappetizing food, too much food offered, food aversions	Nutritional supplements or complete nutritional replacements, including tube feedings or parenteral nutritional support
Systemic illnesses: infection, hepatitis, pancreatitis, malodorous ulcer, endocrinopathies	Zinc, niacin, and vitamin B complex supplements may improve appetite if malnourished
Biochemical effect: hyponatremia, dehydration, hypercalcemia, uremia	
Psychogenic effects: anxiety, depression, fear of vomiting	
Physical complications: fatigue, pain, shortness of breath, chronic obstructive pulmonary disease	
Acquired immune deficiency syndrome (AIDS)	
Food and fluid viewed by the patient as a burden instead of a benefit	
Natural consequences of dying	

FIGURE 2 (continued)

Dietary Management

Do not nag patients to eat. A gentle positive attitude is helpful in encouraging patients to eat. Allow patients to be in charge of their situation; do not criticize them if they eat poorly. If the patient does not eat, remove the food without undue comment.

Serve small servings. A small plate will make the foods more attractive and the serving sizes look smaller and may increase amount of food eaten.

Feed the patient when hungry. Note patient's best meals (usually breakfast is better than supper) and make these the largest meals. Change traditional mealtimes if needed.

Provide the patient's favorite foods.

Contain smells in the kitchen if they cause nausea, vomiting, or anorexia.

Encourage high-calorie foods, including eggnog, milkshake, custard, pudding, peanut butter, cream soups, cheese, fizzy drinks, pie, sherbet, cheesecake. Patients particularly like fresh oranges and freshly prepared lemonade if their mouth is not sore.

Make mealtimes enjoyable; dress to eat, eat at the table, and vary the place of eating.

Other Management

Avoid routine weighing of the patient. Place little emphasis on weight loss. Encourage the patient to wear clothes that fit.

Be sure the patient takes medications appropriately to relieve pain, depression, anxiety, constipation, nausea and vomiting, diarrhea, systemic infections, and biochemical imbalances that may contribute to anorexia.

Encourage mild exercise and relaxation techniques; they may overcome fatigue and sleep problems and improve appetite.

Consider transfusions for anemia which may reduce fatigue and improve appetite.

Consider dental relining if needed and prognosis warrants.

Ameliorate social consequences and physical complications of cachexia. An old photo of the patient without cachexia will help caregivers see the patient as human. A new photo of the cachectic patient with family and friends will help caregivers see the patient as still having a place in the family. A new set of clothes that fit the patient will improve self-esteem.

Note: From: *Nutritional Care of the Terminally III* (pp. 156-158) by C. Gallagher-Allred, 1989, Rockville, MD: Aspen Publishing. Used with permission.

These last mentioned therapies require invasive procedures for placement of catheters or tubes and their effectiveness is limited to situations listed earlier. Their psychological benefit lies in the feeling of "doing something." Since it may be difficult to terminate these interventions once initiated, it is important to carefully explore their burdens and benefits before undertaking them.

Providing Education for Patients/Families and Others

The Hospice Team

The patient and family frequently wish to discuss concerns about the eating problems with various members of the hospice team, not just the nurse and the dietitian. Social workers, chaplains, and volunteers should be provided with information about the physiological aspects of anorexia and cachexia. It is important that they understand the rationale for the medical, nursing, and nutritional management (or possibly non-management) of these problems. Strategies for enhancing oral intake should be highlighted in the volunteer training program. Volunteers as well as the rest of the team should be encouraged to examine their own feelings about food and eating as they work with people who are not eating.

Patients and Family Members

Hospice workers will hear family members say, "I fix his favorite foods and then he won't eat them," or "He must eat if he is to get his strength back." They may not understand or may not want to understand that the loss of appetite is related to the disease. Family members and patients will benefit from an explanation of the physiological basis of the problem.

It is important to explain, in lay terms, that the tumor may be giving off chemicals that cause changes in the perception of taste, and that the satiety or "fullness" center in the brain may also be affected by these chemicals. It is helpful to emphasize that this is a part of the disease and is something over which the patient and family have no control. This explanation may enable the family to shift the blame from the patient to the disease.

Printed Materials

Printed materials can also be helpful. They are useful when shared with family members who cannot be present when the nurse is providing information and they add credibility and reinforcement to verbal instructions. The booklet *Gone From My Sight* (Karnes, 1986) gently suggests that the gradual decrease in eating is a natural part of the dying process. A pamphlet entitled *Nutrition in the Advanced Cancer Patient* (North Hospice, 1991) prepared by the North Hospice staff explains the physiological basis of eating problems, offers practical suggestions for improving intake, acknowledges the emotions evoked by the loss, and it suggests strategies for coping with feelings around this loss.

Helping Families Cope with the Emotional Aspects of the Loss

While education is effective in dealing with misinformation about anorexia, cachexia, and malnutrition, the feelings of fear, anger, frustration, and sadness are more difficult to assuage. The most important function for all members of the team is to provide a listening ear. Much family frustration is born out of a sense of helplessness with the inability to "do something" for the patient. Family may be guided to find non-food ways of caregiving or nurturing. Suggestions might include reading to the patient, doing a manicure, or administering gentle massage of the feet, hands, or head.

The sense of loss may be most profound for the family member who had been the food preparer. This person has lost a role, a source of self-esteem and, perhaps, an enjoyable and comfortable pasttime. This person should be counseled to explore feelings about the personal aspects of this loss. The person may benefit from receiving permission and encouragement to practice self-care activities such as eating out with friends or cooking at a shelter kitchen one afternoon a week.

Patients often report they eat because they feel pressured to by family members. When a patient chooses not to, but more likely cannot eat, family should be helped to honor the preference. Encouraging family to share their feelings of frustration with the hospice team, rather than with the patient, will relieve this pressure and will improve the patient's quality of life. Patients should be empowered to be in charge of the foods and fluids served to them.

DEHYDRATION IN THE IMMINENTLY DYING

The issue of fluid intake is imbued with much of the same emotion as is the eating and feeding of solid foods. The parent of an ill child is admonished to give plenty of fluids. Similarly, the novice nurse is schooled in the benefits of forcing fluids. Throughout the medical and lay worlds the term dehydration refers to a negative state; a condition calling out for correction. There are ill effects from dehydration (Brooker, 1992) (see Figure 3). The most apparent, and the most distressing for patient and family alike, is that of dry mucosa. Nausea, vomiting, neuromuscular irritability, restlessness, and a diminished level of consciousness may also accompany dehydration (Zerwekh, 1983).

On the other hand, dehydration is also a normal part of the physiology of dying. Dying cancer patients may become dehydrated for a variety of reasons among them nausea and vomiting, diarrhea, bowel obstruction, and bleeding. They also have reduced oral intake due to a deteriorating level of consciousness and to the simple loss of desire to take fluids. Billings (1985) suggests that the latter is a disorder in thirst perception.

Prior to the middle of this century, medical science lacked any technology to correct dehydration, but now intravenous lines and nasogastric tubes are commonplace. The availability of a technology, however, does not *a priori* mean that a patient's situation will be improved by its use. In palliative care hydration therapy may impose more burdens than benefits (Andrews & Levine, 1989). When making decisions about the use of artificial hydration, the guiding concern should be whether it will contribute to the patient's comfort.

Beneficial Effects of Dehydration in the Terminally Ill

The positive effects of the natural process of dehydration in the imminently dying are worth factoring into the decisions related to

FIGURE 3. Dehydration: Effects on People with Terminal Illness

Symptom	Physiological Basis	Nursing Care
1. Thirst	Cells shrink stimulating 'thirst osmoreceptors' in hypothalamus	Mouth care to ease discomfort and prevent infection. Ice chips. Oral intake as tolerated.
2. Dry, inelastic skin	Loss of normal elasticity– cells 'dry out'	Soft mattress, careful lifting and turns to prevent skin damage. Care with IV sites. No soap. Assess lethargy and resultant immobility.
3. Temperature increase	Regulations of body temperature disturbed. Normal temperature control requires 800ml fluid intake daily.	Monitoring of temperature as at risk of infection. Skin care. Cool wipes. Fan. Cool drinks. Light clothing/ bedcovers.
4. Increased viscosity of secretions	Extracellular fluid (ECF) deficit	Deep breathing/ coughing exercises and physiotherapy if necessary/tolerated.
5. Postural hypotension	Decreased plasma volume, decreased circulating blood flow and inability to compensate	Monitor ambulation closely. Observe for weakness, dizziness, faints.
6. Increased drug toxicity	Mainly affects kidneys. Decreased blood volume causes increased concentration of drugs	Monitor for side-effects of particular drug administered. Minimize medications prescribed.
7. Apprehension/ restlessness	Cellular dehydration in brain due to shift of water from cells to ECF compartment	Monitor levels of anxiety and ability to function adequately. Assess safety.

Reproduced by kind permission of *Nursing Times* where this table first appreared in the article "Dehydration Before Death" on January 8th, 1992.

providing artificial hydration. Musgrave (1990) and Zerwekh (1983) cite the following beneficial effects of dehydration:

- Decreased urine output resulting in less incontinence and less need for toileting,
- Decreased production of gastric fluids resulting in less nausea and vomiting,
- Decreased pulmonary secretions resulting in less need for suctioning,
- Diminished incidence of edema and ascites.

It also has been noted by those who work with the dying that there is a lessened need for analgesia as the patient becomes more dehydrated. While the etiology of this phenomenon is speculative, Printz (1988) summarizes the physiologic explanations. They include: (1) alterations in the metabolic state leading to a decreased level of consciousness ranging from lethargy to coma; (2) ketone accumulation causing loss of sensation, resulting from caloric deprivation; and (3) increased production of opioid peptides or endorphins when the body is in a state of water deprivation or fasting. Whatever the explanation for this phenomenon, staff should feel comfortable in reassuring families that, not only is dehydration not a painful condition, but state of dehydration before death may even cause the patient to perceive less pain.

The Burdens of Hydration Therapy

Among the burdens of hydration therapy are the need for invasive and often uncomfortable tubes and needles. When the patient is being cared for at home, it is necessary to consider the ability of the family to manage tubes and pumps. Although some families will welcome the task, viewing even the artificial intervention as a means of feeding and nurturing; others will not be able to manage it; and still others will see it as disturbingly invasive as well as being futile. Also to be considered are the detrimental effects of potential fluid overload (Brooker, 1992), which are arrayed in Figure 4.

FIGURE 4. Effects of Fluid Overload

Symptom	Physiological Basis	Nursing Care
l. Oedema	Increased ECF causing decreased blood flow to skin surface by pressure on arterial micro-circulation	Soft mattress, avoid sharp objects. Care with injections. Safety to prevent skin damage. Care of all pressure areas.
2. Increased urinary output	Release of ADH inhibited	Catheterization if incontinent and mobility impaired to prevent skin damage. Increased use of bedpan/commode causing increased effort, assistance may be required. Skin care. Barrier cream. Maintain dignity.
3. Pulmonary oedema/ increased respiratory secretion	Increased ECF volume	Suction if unable to expectorate. Coughing, deep breathing with emphasis on expiration. Turning to reduce feeling of 'choking' or 'drowning.' Medical intervention.
4. Increased gastrointestinal secretions	Increased ECF volume	Nasogastric tube if vomiting. Monitor for ascites, also for any pain from oedema causing pressure on tumour present. Antiemetics.
5. Twitching, hyper- irritability, mental disturbances, convulsions, coma	Possible cerebral oedema	Monitor degree of mental disturbances and so on. Symptomatic relief. Safety. Care of significant others. Relaxation techniques.

Reproduced by kind permission of *Nursing Times* where this table first appeared in the article "Dehydration Before Death" on January 8th, 1992.

Assessment of the Patient and Family

Once it has been established that the patient is dehydrated and cannot maintain an adequate oral intake, the nurse, the dietitian, the physician, and the patient and family need to collaborate about whether or not to intervene. The following factors may guide decision-making: (1) Prognosis. Is the patient near death and is the dehydration part of the dying process, or might this person live for weeks with an improved quality of life with correction of the dehydration? (2) The patient's wishes. Hydration therapy requires either an inpatient admission or intensive home care management. Is the patient willing to be subjected to needles, pumps, bags, and strangers in the home? (3) The family's desires and abilities. Is the family able and willing to manage their responsibilities in managing a home infusion? The nurse, dietitian, and physician should lead the patient and family through an examination of the burdens and benefits of this treatment.

Suggesting Appropriate Interventions

While dehydration is not uncommon at the time of death, medical, nursing and dietary efforts should be made to prevent its premature onset. Medical management of nausea, vomiting and diarrhea should be aggressive. Dietary efforts to enhance oral fluid intake should be made as long as the patient wishes and can tolerate them.

Aggressive management with intravenous fluids should be instituted only after consideration of the previously-mentioned factors. Hospice programs must employ staff or make arrangements with an agency that is competent to administer home intravenous therapy. Education and support are needed to minimize the burden on the family caregiving system in the home.

Should the decision be made to not correct the condition, interventions must be aimed at minimizing the ill effects of dehydration. Gallagher-Allred (1989) presents appropriate therapeutic suggestions for management of dehydration (see Figure 5).

In addition to her suggestions, our staff at North Hospice has found commercially available lubricants, artificial tears, and saliva to be of help. Family members may be more distressed than the patient by the dry mucosa. Therefore, meticulous and frequent oral care is essential. Ice chips and sips of fluids should be offered as long as the patient is able to swallow. Tranquilizing medications may be used to combat restlessness and muscular twitching.

Providing Education for Patients/Families and Others

The Healthcare Team

Health care professionals may be under the influence of the same myths about dehydration as is the general public. To medical and nursing students, dehydration is seen as a symptom in need of reversal. Rarely is terminal dehydration a subject of academic discussion. Palliative care professionals are obligated to provide education on this topic. Relationships should be established with medical schools and residency programs whenever possible. Sharing some of the current literature and observations from your clinical experience may be of use when working with health professionals who feel obligated to always treat dehydration.

The Patient and the Family

The most effective means of avoiding unnecessary intervention is to provide education to the patient and family. A family that is aware of the inevitability of dehydration problems at the end of life is less likely to request intervention. The nurse should be prepared to clearly outline the burdens and the benefits in lay terms.

Helping Families Cope with the Emotional Aspects of the Loss

Many families seem comforted when it is pointed out to them that dehydration is a natural part of the dying process and that it has beneficial effects for the patient. They also seem to appreciate the idea that it has only been within the last forty years that reversal of this normal process has been attempted. Some families will wish to do everything possible even if the intervention gives only the illusion of prolonging their loved one's life.

FIGURE 5. The Management of Dehydration

Symptoms and Cause of Symptoms	Drug Management
Reduced intake of fluids due to inability to consume liquids: comatose, weakness, inability to swallow	To moisten lips, try Vaseline, Chap Stick, or K-Y jelly
Excessive fluid losses due to: excess sweating fever nausea and vomiting diarrhea fistula and ostomy losses excess urine output deficiency of antidiuretic hormone	To moisten mouth, use mouth rinses; avoid the drying effects of lemon and glycerin. Remove debris in mouth with frequent dilute peroxide and water rinses
	Treat mouth infections appropriately
Electrolyte imbalances due to: kidney failure catabolism liver failure	Manage electrolyte imbalance secondary to endocrine problems with hormone replacement and other medications as appropriate
	Consider IV fluid replacement
	Treat nausea and vomiting with antiemetics

Discontinuing therapies once they have been started has emotional ramifications. Shannon (1987) addresses the idea that initiating a therapy is tantamount to making a commitment to the patient's recovery and that admitting that the therapy is not working can be difficult. He also suggests that neither the medical profession nor the family is obligated to continue treatments that are not achieving the goals of therapy. Possessing knowledge of that fact and feeling comfortable with it, however, do not always go hand in hand.

For the family struggling with decision-making, it might be helpful to point out that a time-limited trial offers the assurance that everything has been tried. It should also be pointed out that it is not illegal or immoral or unethical to withdraw medical treatments that are not effective. The family may feel less burdened if the hospice

Figure 5 (continued)

Dietary Management

Encourage liquids and favorite beverages, such as ice chips, juices, carbonated beverages, gelatin, sherbet, and broth-based soups

Encourage milk, milkshakes, creamed soups, and eggnogs if mucus or fever is not problematic

Be creative: try carbonated beverage ice cubes and popsicles of juice and Polycose

Discuss goals, expectations, and quality of life issues with patient, family, and health care team when considering tube feedings or parenteral feedings for treatment of dehydration or electrolyte imbalance

Other Management

Treat underlying renal failure with dialysis, liver failure with shunts, and catabolism if appropriate

Reduce ambient room temperature or provide lighter bed clothes and blankets if excessive sweating

Note: From: *Nutritional Care of the Terminally Ill* (pp. 164-165) by C. Gallagher-Allred, 1989, Rockville, MD: Aspen Publishing. Used with permission.

team characterizes food and fluids as medical treatments that are no longer indicated if they are not improving the patient's condition. Gradually reducing the fluid administration rate, instead of suddenly discontinuing the fluids, may be a more comfortable strategy for some families. Families should also be informed that discontinuing intravenous fluids will not result in the patient's immediate death and that, in fact, dying patients may live days to weeks without a source of fluids.

CONCLUDING THOUGHTS

Cancer patients and their family members must cope with multiple losses as the disease progresses. The lost ability to eat and drink is a real and perceived harbinger of the ultimate loss—death.

While anorexia and cachexia are normal parts of the clinical picture in an advancing malignancy, often the loss of a patient's ability to eat and drink will not be easily accepted by the family. Because this loss has profound emotional, spiritual, and physical ramifications, it is important that an interdisciplinary team help patients and families cope with this difficult problem.

REFERENCES

Amenta, M. O., & Bohnet, N. L. (1986). *Nursing care of the terminally ill.* Boston: Little, Brown and Company.

Andrews, M. R., & Levine, A. M. (1989). Dehydration in the terminal patient: Perceptions of hospice nurses. *American Journal of Hospice Care,* 6(1), 31-34.

Bernstein, I. L. (1986). Etiology of anorexia in cancer. *Cancer,* 58, 1881-1886.

Billings, J. A. (1985). Comfort measures for the terminally ill: Is dehydration painful? *American Journal of the Geriatric Society,* 33(11), 808-810.

Brooker, S. (1992). Dehydration before death. *Nursing Times,* 88(2) 59-62.

Bruera, E., & MacDonald, R. N. (1988). Nutrition in cancer patients: An update and review of our experience. *Journal of Pain and Symptom Management,* 3(3), 133-140.

Gallagher-Allred, C. (1989). *Nutritional care of the terminally ill.* Rockville, MD: Aspen.

Holden, C. (1991). Anorexia in the terminally ill cancer patient: The emotional impact on the patient and the family. *The Hospice Journal,* 7(3), 73-84.

Karnes, B. (1986). *Gone from my sight.* (P.O. Box 335, Stilwell, KS 66085).

Kaye, P. (1990). *Symptom control in hospice and palliative care.* Essex, CT: Hospice Education Institute.

Musgrave, C. F. (1990). Terminal dehydration: To give or not to give intravenous fluids? *Cancer Nursing,* 13(1), 62-66.

National Cancer Institute. (1987). *Eating hints: Recipes and tips for better nutrition during cancer treatment.* (NIH Publication No. 87-2079). U.S. Department of Health and Human Services, Bethesda, MD.

North Hospice. (1991). *Nutrition in the advanced cancer patient.* Robbinsdale, MN.

Ohnuma, T. (1989). Nutritional support of cancer patients during cancer progression. In P.V. Wooley (Ed.), *Cancer management in man: Biological response modifiers, chemotherapy, antibiotics, hyperthermia, supporting measures.* Netherlands: Kluwer Academic Publishers.

Printz, L. A. (1988). Is withholding hydration a valid comfort measure in the terminally ill? *Geriatrics,* 43(11), 84-88.

Shannon, T. A. (1987). *Let them go free.* Kansas City, MO: Sheed and Ward.

Shika, M., & Brennan, M. F. (1989). Supportive care of the cancer patient. In V.

DeVita, S. Hellman, S. Rosenberg (Eds.), *Cancer: Principles and practice of oncology* (3rd ed.). Philadelphia: J. B. Lippincott.

Simonetti, J. (1985). National survey conducted by American Journal of Hospice Care. *American Journal of Hospice Care, 2*(5), 12.

Souba, W. W., & Copeland, E. M. (1989). Hyperalimentation in cancer. *CAA Cancer Journal for Clinicians, 39,* 105-113.

Torosian, M., & Daly, J. (1986). Nutritional support in the cancer-bearing host. *Cancer, 58,* 1915-1929.

Wachtel, T., Allen-Masterson, S., Reuben, D., Goldberg, R., & Mor, V. (1988). The end stage cancer patient: Terminal common pathway. *The Hospice Journal, 4*(4), 43-80.

Warren, S. (1932). The immediate cause of death in cancer. *American Journal of Medical Sciences, 68,* 683-690.

Zerwekh, J. V. (1983). The dehydration question. *Nursing, 13*(1), 47-51.

Nutritional Care
of the Terminally Ill Adult

Julie O'Sullivan Maillet
Dorothy King

SUMMARY. Nutrition and hydration options are based on many considerations that arise during the various phases of the dying process. This paper includes discussion of the psychological issues affecting intake, assessment techniques to determine whether nutrient intake is adequate, feeding suggestions for the caregiving family, and some guidelines for routine and complex care of the terminally ill adult. The ultimate goal is to improve quality of life for each terminally ill individual through a focus on patient benefit and patient care.

INTRODUCTION

The overarching goals in palliative nutrition care for the terminal stage of life are to maximize the patient's nutritional benefit, pleasure, and comfort from food while minimizing discomfort. The

Julie O'Sullivan Maillet, PhD, RD, is Associate Professor and Chairman, Department of Primary Care, School of Health Related Professions, University of Medicine and Dentistry of New Jersey. Dorothy King, PhD, RD, is a nutrition consultant in New York, NY.

Address correspondence to: Julie O'Sullivan Maillet, PhD, RD, Department of Primary Care, School of Health Related Professions, University of Medicine and Dentistry of New Jersey, 65 Bergen St., Newark, NJ 07107-3001.

[Haworth co-indexing entry note]: "Nutritional Care of the Terminally Ill Adult." Maillet, Julie O'Sullivan and Dorothy King. Co-published simultaneously in *The Hospice Journal* (The Haworth Press, Inc.) Vol. 9, Nos. 2/3, 1993, pp. 37-54: and: *Nutrition and Hydration in Hospice Care: Needs, Strategies, Ethics* (eds: Gallagher-Allred, Charlette, and Madalon O'Rawe Amenta) The Haworth Press, Inc., 1993, pp. 37-54. Multiple copies of this article/chapter may be purchased from The Haworth Document Delivery Center [1-800-3-HAWORTH; 9:00 a.m. - 5:00 p.m. (EST)].

© 1993 by The Haworth Press, Inc. All rights reserved.

37

common discomforts–all contributing to decreased food and fluid intake as well as to decreased nutrient absorption–might include pain, shortness of breath, depression, weakness, anorexia, vomiting, diarrhea, and gastro-intestinal obstructions.

Another important goal is to deal with the fallout from prominent media presentations that have heightened the nutrition fears of patients and families. They fear being coerced and/or force fed at one extreme and/or being starved by cavalier, passive neglect at the other. Developing ethical, humanitarian feeding guidelines requires wisdom and deliberation in seeking that delicate balance between too much and too little. Weighing all the crucial factors and establishing what is appropriate for each patient under changing physical and environmental conditions during the various phases of the dying process are the challenges.

This paper discusses some of the components of coordinating interdisciplinary hospice team information and services for the creation and implementation of individualized, appropriate nutrition care plans for the terminally ill adult. We emphasize the dietitian's special professional responsibility in managing the who (patient/family), the what (symptoms), the where (care setting), and the by whom (family, staff, volunteer).

THE ROLE OF THE HOSPICE DIETITIAN

The unique professional role and responsibility of the registered dietitian is to provide expert consultation to patient, family, and staff on the creative variety of feasible options that might meet each individual patient's evolving nutrient needs while catering to the patient's food preferences and tolerances. The dietitian deals with oral diets with or without therapeutic modifications, oral supplements, and enteral and parenteral nutrition. "No individual [professional] is better qualified to interpret and coordinate . . . nutrition issues. Who needs the hospice dietitian? The patient, family and health care team do" (Gallagher-Allred, 1985, p. 11).

Terminally ill patients and their families need honest, open communication about what nutrition and feeding can do. They also need the free exchange of questions and answers about the best possible nutrition care and available resources. Common questions include the relationship between intake and symptom management, and the symptoms that may result from not eating. Assurances that food intake and abandonment are not linked, with the emphasis on affection not food, is often essential for the family. The hospice team needs to acknowledge and support patients' rights to make both small food choices and major life choices pertaining to nutrient intake (Gallagher-Allred, 1989).

"It is the dietitian's responsibility to provide a combination of emotional support and technical nutrition advice on how to best achieve each patient's goals within legal parameters" (American Dietetic Association [ADA], 1992, p. 996). The dietitian assesses patient nutritional status affected by disease, treatment, and other physiological determinants, and constructs a creative plan of feasible feeding alternatives. In order to ensure emotional and physical acceptability, patient preferences and the minimization of food aversions and intolerances are given high priority.

Liberalization and elimination of rigid, long standing dietary restrictions based on rationales for prevention or treatment of chronic disease are advocated except when they cause physical discomfort. For example, cholesterol restrictions are directed toward potential long term cardiovascular benefits. Continued elimination of eggs may be counterproductive in the diet of the terminally ill because eggs are an inexpensive, high protein, densely nutritious food, soft and easy to swallow, and easy to prepare.

The majority of hospice patients have cancer as a primary diagnosis. As a result of previous cancer therapies such as surgery, chemotherapy, or radiation, it is estimated that 60% to 80% of these patients require minor diet modification in order to achieve comfort in eating and digesting (Gallagher-Allred, 1985). The hospice dietitian optimizes the variety in food choices by the frequent updating of symptoms and she or he experiments with what works for each patient as the patient's condition fluctuates. There may be bad days or segments of days when little can be taken orally. At other times a diet free of restrictions may be copiously consumed and enjoyed. This course, rarely linear, usually assumes a zig zag pattern (Bloch, 1990).

THE MEANING OF ENTERAL
AND PARENTERAL NUTRITION

In the area of enteral and parenteral nutrition, feeding can be a powerful symbol of hope. Although the infusion of nutrients may not enhance physical strength to a measurable degree, if it helps the patient psychologically it may be viewed as a form of pain medication. At times, basic tubefeeding that alleviates anxiety due to poor food intake, may so enhance patient/family interaction that the simple fact of feeding improves quality of life. The value of moderating the appearance of cachexia, having the patient once again "looking good," may add to the patient's sense of dignity, and help to keep the family comfortable.

The provision of nutrition and hydration, then, can be considered a nonmedical as well as a medical treatment. In either case it is the patient's and family's values and beliefs rather than those of the health professionals that must take precedence. That means supporting patients' and families' decisions. Advancement to tubefeeding can be considered invasive, extraordinary, and heroic care to the patient who feels that the tube feeding detracts from his or her dignity. To another patient and/or family the neglect of tubefeeding as an option may cause feelings of hopelessness and abandonment.

GUIDELINES FOR ROUTINE AND COMPLEX CARE

For routine care, the feeding and hydration preferences of the patient should be determined when care begins. Interdisciplinary team communication, with the patient at the center of the team, is necessary in the discussion of feeding alternatives. The patient's nutrient needs in relation to his/her nutrient intake must be continually evaluated so that the dietitian can identify the feeding options, the benefits and burdens of liberalizing previous diet restrictions, and the need for assistance in the delivery of meals. Access to food and the strength to prepare meals should be analyzed. The purchasing of prepared foods, such as frozen dinners, may reduce the chances of malnutrition. In addition, the use of governmental and private home delivered meal programs can foster intake of nutritionally balanced meals. A social worker often has access to this information.

Taste and smell acuity in the terminally ill vary from intense to diminished. Types of food and sites of preparation, therefore, should be managed accordingly. Patients and families need to understand anorexia. They need to understand that the patient may refuse favorite foods because of alterations in his or her sense of taste and smell. The hospice team, especially the dietitian, may need to help the family understand that a hot nourishing meal may not be what the patient can benefit from at certain times, that offering any foods the patient requests when the patient asks for them may be the more useful approach.

Assessment of Nutritional Status

Signs of dehydration and malnutrition may be subtle, so the care provider must make a conscious effort to watch for clues (The Hastings Center, 1987). These include swallowing difficulties, limited intake, and evidence of wasting: weight loss, loosened clothes, loss of skin turgor. Because physical symptoms may be affected by medications, and edema may mask actual weight loss, the observer must be meticulous in his or her examination. And because the gross clinical manifestations of nutritional deficit are the last signs of the deficiency–reserves become exhausted first, then biochemical and clinical functions become compromised–it is paramount that the caregiver provide ongoing monitoring of signs of inadequate food availability and intake. Amount of food purchased in a week, lack of variety of foods, and large portions left on the plate are indications of increased vulnerability to nutritional problems. A model nutritional assessment protocol appears as Figure 1.

Malnutrition decreases strength and the sense of well being. Thus food and nutrients, if they can be tolerated, should be encouraged until death is imminent.

Symptom Management

Optimal nutrition and hydration are the basis for maximizing physical strength and well being, preventing dehydration, hunger,

FIGURE 1. Nutrition Assessment Form

Patient Symptoms

1.   Does the patient have any of the following symptoms?

* nausea   No _____   Yes _____
* vomiting   No _____   Yes _____

If yes, is nausea and/or vomiting associated with: (check all that apply)

* meals   No _____   Yes _____
* lack of meals   No _____   Yes _____
* taste of foods (sweet,   No _____   Yes _____
  spicy tart, salty, bland,
  protein-containing)
* sight, smell of particular   No _____   Yes _____
  foods
* temperature of foods   No _____   Yes _____
  (hot, cold)
* depression, anxiety?   No _____   Yes _____
* any conditioned response   No _____   Yes _____
  e.g. modification box,
  perfume, thoughts of
  doctor's office,
  abdominal pain, etc.?
* mouth sores   No _____   Yes _____
* dry mouth   No _____   Yes _____
* drooling   No _____   Yes _____
* ill-fitting dentures   No _____   Yes _____
* inability to chew   No _____   Yes _____
  properly
* inability to swallow   No _____   Yes _____
  easily
* diarrhea   No _____   Yes _____
* constipation   No _____   Yes _____
* fluid accumulation   No _____   Yes _____
* dehydration   No _____   Yes _____

FIGURE 1 (continued)

2. Does the patient have any of the following conditions?

- colostomy   No _____   Yes _____
- urinary catheter   No _____   Yes _____

  if either present, is   No _____   Yes _____
  what you eat modified
  to influence elimination?

- functioning GI feeding   No _____   Yes _____
  or drainage tube
- functioning IV feeding   No _____   Yes _____
  or hydration line
- How is the patient's appetite?

  - always good   No _____   Yes _____
  - usually, but not   No _____   Yes _____
    always pretty good
  - have to force   No _____   Yes _____
    food to eat
  - cannot stand the   No _____   Yes _____
    thought of food

Simple Dietary History

1. Is eating a pleasurable experience?   No _____   Yes _____

2. Could it be more pleasurable?   No _____   Yes _____

3. Are there any foods that you do   No _____   Yes _____
   not like or avoid? If so, what?

4. Are you allergic or intolerant to   No _____   Yes _____
   any foods? If so, what?

5. Do you have any cultural or religious   No _____   Yes _____
   food preferences?

6. Have you developed any food changes   No _____   Yes _____
   since being ill?

7. If appropriate, obtain a dietary history including:
   - when, what, how much, where, and with whom the patient eats during the
     day

8. Do you take any vitamin/mineral   No _____   Yes _____
   supplements?

   If so, what?

FIGURE 1 (continued)

9. If appropriate, try to determine the following:
    - average daily intake of
        1. kilocalories
        2. fluid
        3. fiber
        4. alcohol

10. Weight Change
    - Has your weight basically been   No _____ Yes _____
      stable?
      If no, what is current weight? _____
        - What was typical weight? _____
        - Has your clothing size changed? If yes, how? _____
    - Does this weight change concern you?   No _____ Yes _____
    - Was this weight change intentional?   No _____ Yes _____
    - Does this weight change make you   No _____ Yes _____
      more dependent on others?
      If so, how?
      If so, does it bother you?   No _____ Yes _____
    - If we can, do you want us to try   No _____ Yes _____
      to do something about your weight?

Ability to Eat and Progression of Diet

    - Do you find it difficult to let   No _____ Yes _____
      others feed you?
    - Do you find it difficult to let others   No _____ Yes _____
      shop, cook, or clean up for you?
    - Do you need more assistance in   No _____ Yes _____
      shopping, cooking, or cleaning up?
    - To the respiratory troubled patient   No _____ Yes _____
      if appropriate: Do you sometimes
      feel you'll drown or choke to death if
      you drink or eat?
    - Have you tried supplemental-nutrient   No _____ Yes _____
      dense drinks?
    - Would you be willing to try them again?   No _____ Yes _____
    - If you become unable or find it   No _____ Yes _____
      undesirable to eat or drink, would
      you want to be given fluids by vein?

FIGURE 1 (continued)

To be fed by tube into your stomach?   No _____ Yes _____
To be fed nutrients by vein?   No _____ Yes _____
• Do you have an advance directive?   No _____ Yes _____

Family Concerns

1. Ask the caregiver(s) questions, such as:
   • How well do you think the patient is eating?
   Good _____   Fair _____   Poor _____
   • Are the amount and variety the patient eats acceptable to you?
   No _____   Yes _____
   • Is there anything you would like to tell the patient or express to me about the patient's eating that concerns the patient or concerns you?
   No _____   Yes _____

   If so, what?
   • Are there community services I can facilitate access to for you, such as Meals on Wheels, food stamps, or commercial nutritional supplements?
   No _____   Yes _____

   If so, what?

Summary

1. Symptoms suggest potential difficulties with intake?   No _____ Yes _____
2. Weight or weight change suggest nutritional risk?   No _____ Yes _____
3. The diet history suggests deficiencies in nutrient intake?   No _____ Yes _____
4. Patient may need help with feeding.   No _____ Yes _____
   Obtaining food.   No _____ Yes _____
5. Patient wants:
   supplemental feeding   No _____ Yes _____
   IV Fluids   No _____ Yes _____
   tubefeedings, if needed   No _____ Yes _____
   parenteral feeding if needed   No _____ Yes _____
6. Family has concerns.   No _____ Yes _____

Adapted, with permission, from: Gallagher-Allred, C. (1989). *Nutritional Care of the Terminally Ill.* pp. 120-123. Rockville, MD: Aspen Publishers, Inc.

thirst, and potential nutrient deficiencies. As stated previously, achievement of optimal nutrition is based on individual patient need. Has gastrointestinal ingestion, digestion, absorption, or elimination been altered? Has the dying process slowed gastric emptying resulting in decreased hunger? Are treatments or medications causing side effects? Has dysphagia increased the fear of choking? Table 1 provides dietary guidelines for the treatment of several symptoms such as constipation, diarrhea, mouth problems, nausea, and vomiting. The need to tailor the guidelines to the individual to meet specific physical and emotional needs and desires cannot be overemphasized. In all instances, the individual patient's response to treatment of symptoms should be respected.

The Sequence of Feedings

At the point that nutritional intake and hydration become marginal, the first question is whether enteral or parenteral nutrition or hydration will sustain or decrease the quality of life. Before that question is asked, however, every effort should be made to enhance oral intake. The following suggestions may be helpful: offer small frequent feedings of easy to ingest foods or commercial nutritional supplements; provide assistance in the feeding process; and have easily available calorically dense foods and beverages on hand. When and if these measures are ineffective and the quality of life question has been answered, tubefeeding or parenteral feeding may be considered. The maxim: When in doubt *feed*.

Hunger and Thirst

When death is imminent the patient may lose all desire to take anything by mouth, and the pushing of fluids and foods in any case will have no real benefit (National Conference of Catholic Bishops' Committee, 1992). Malnutrition and dehydration feel different than hunger and thirst. "Medical procedures for supplying nutrition and hydration treat malnutrition and dehydration; they may or may not relieve hunger and thirst. Conversely hunger and thirst can be treated without necessarily using medical nutrition and hydration techniques and without necessarily correcting dehydration or malnourishment" (The Hastings Center, 1987, p. 59-60). For example, thirst can be relieved by ice chips and moistening the mouth without correcting the dehydration. In addition, " . . . patients in their last days before death may spontaneously reduce their intake of nutrition and hydration without experiencing hunger and thirst" (The Hastings Center, 1987, p. 60).

Therefore, the decision to medically nourish or hydrate must be made on an individual benefit/risk basis. The possibilities range from feeding enterally or parenterally to foregoing feeding altogether. The risk or burden to patient/family from enteral or parenteral feeding may be too physically or psychologically painful, too restrictive as in the case of forcing hospitalization, or too expensive.

Advance Directives

An advance directive indicating preferences for or against artificial nutrition is useful both in assistance in decision making and in validation of the authenticity of the current option of the individual. Under specific irreversible conditions of decisional incapacity, the staff and family are obligated to honor the patient's wishes (directive); the patient has the right to alter the advance directive.

ETHICS: TO FEED OR NOT TO FEED

The ethics of patient care, especially in palliative care, can present difficult nutrition decisions and dilemmas. Intuition and principles may clash, varying traditions and histories may alter the viewpoints of patients and caregivers. Nonetheless, patients and caregivers must decide hydration and nutrition questions daily. Caregivers need to recognize and deal with their own personal biases and respect patients' uncoerced, informed decisions.

The last decade has produced much debate among medical, legal, and religious scholars on the emotionally charged question of whether enteral tube feedings and parenteral nutrition support are ethically comparable to other medically-supplied life-sustaining procedures such as ventilator support. The debate gives rise to two questions, are enteral and parenteral feedings optional heroic med-

TABLE 1. Dietary Management of Common Symptoms in Terminally Ill Patients

Belching
- Try to determine which foods cause the belching especially the gas producers: carbonated drinks, beer and alcohol, dairy products, other high fat foods, and legumes and vegetables high in fiber. Let the patient make all final choices about what to and what not to eat.
- Have the patient eat solids at mealtime and take fluids between meals, not with solid foods.
- Have the patient eat slowly and relax before, during, and after eating. The patient should not, however, recline just after eating.
- The patient should to the degree possible keep his or her mouth closed when chewing or swallowing, not chew gum, and not suck through straws.

Constipation
- If adequate fluid intake can be maintained, the patient should eat high fiber foods–whole grains, nuts, vegetables and fruits such as pineapple, prunes, and raisins. If severe constipation, dehydration, or obstruction become problems high fiber foods should be avoided.
- If they contribute to constipation, discontinue calcium and iron supplements, and limit cheeses and rich desserts.
- Have the patient increase his or her fluid intake to maximum tolerable levels. This is especially important if bulk-forming laxatives are being used. Offer cider, fruit juices, and prune juice. An effective, low cost laxative: 1-2 ounces with the evening meal of a mixture of two cups applesauce, two cups unprocessed bran, and one cup 100% prune juice.

Diarrhea
- If they are contributing to the diarrhea, urge the limitation of foods such as milk and ice cream; whole grain products; nuts and legumes; greens, raw and gas-forming vegetables; fruits with seeds and skins; fresh pineapple and raisins; alcohol and caffeine containing beverages.
- Urge the patient to eat bananas, apple sauce, peeled apples, tapioca, rice, peanut butter, refined grains, crackers, pasta, cream of wheat, oatmeal, and cooked vegetables.
- Encourage eating the meal without liquids. Offer fluids, especially those containing sugar and electrolytes, an hour after eating.
- Have the patient relax before, during, and after a meal.
- If dehydration accompanies the diarrhea, offer foods high in potassium.
- With AIDS patients, enteral and/or parenteral nutritional support may be appropriate. In such cases the diet formula should be high in calories and protein, and low in fiber.

Hypercalcemia
- Do not discourage foods with a high calcium content, such as ice cream, if the patient wants them; but caution against the use of calcium and vitamin D supplements.
- Encourage fluids as tolerated, particularly carbonated drinks containing phosphoric acid.

Mental Disorders
- Urge the patient to discontinue alcohol and foods and beverages high in caffeine -- coffee, tea, chocolate -- if they contribute to anxiety, sleep deprivation, or depression.
- With the *drowsy or apathetic* patient help the family to assume the responsibility for feeding him or her. Urge them to prepare the patient's favorite foods in bite sizes and/or soft forms if the patient can be helped to spoon feed him- or herself. Help the family protect the patient and others from possible harm that might be inflicted by the patient by shutting off stoves or removing knobs, removing matches, and locking doors to cupboards that contain alcohol, medications, or poisons. Unplug microwave ovens and put away small electrical appliances.
- Urge the family to be cautious when hand feeding the *agitated or confused* patient: feed with a spoon and do not allow patient to handle utensils. Use reality orientation by reminding the patient what time of day it is, what meal is being served, and that the foods being served are his or her favorites. While trying to make mealtime pleasant by reminiscing about the past, minimize conversation if the patient appears frightened or confused. Urge the family to carefully consider the pros and cons of waking the patient if he or she is asleep at mealtime.
- In the case of the *stuporous or comatose* patient, remind the family that semi-starvation and dehydration are not painful to the patient and, if they ask about it, explore with them the pros and cons of enteral and parenteral nutritional support.

Mouth Problems
- When foods taste *bitter* to the patient -- instead of the foods usually associated with bitter tastes: red meats, sour juices, tomatoes, coffee and tea, chocolate -- suggest that he or she try poultry, fish, dairy products and eggs. Do not serve foods in metallic containers or use metallic utensils. Use herbs and spices as seasoning and encourage sweet fruit drinks, ice lollipops, and carbonated beverages.
- When foods taste *too sweet* to the patient, encourage the drinking of sour juices; cooking with lemon juice, vinegar, spices, herbs, and mint; add pickles when appropriate.

- When foods have *no taste* for the patient suggest marination, if approprate; the serving of highly seasoned foods; the addition of sugar; and serving foods at room temperature.
- When the patient has *difficulty swallowing* urge frequent small meals of soft or pureed foods; caution against foods that might irritate the mouth or esophagus, such as acidic fruits or juices; foods that are spicy or very hot or cold, alcohol, and carbonated beverages.
- When the patient has *mouth sores* urge cold and blenderized foods, cream soups and gravies, eggnog, milkshakes, cheesecake and cream pies, and macaroni and cheese. Have the patient avoid alcohol, and acidic, spicy, rough, hot, and highly salted foods.
- When the patient has a *dry mouth* urge frequent sips of water, juice, ice chips, ice lollipops, ice cream, fruitades, or slushy-frozen baby foods mixed with fruit juices. Suggest sucking on hard candies to stimulate saliva production. Solid foods should be moist, pureed if necessary, and not too tart, too hot, or too cold.

Nausea and Vomiting

- Suggest that the patient not eat.
- If the patient wants to and can tolerate eating, encourage small meals of cool, odor-free foods. Avoid fatty or greasy and fried foods; avoid high bulk foods; do not mix hot and cold foods at the same meal. Discourage the intake of alcohol, and sweet and/or spicy foods.
- Urge the patient to eat slowly and avoid overeating, to relax before and after meals, and to avoid physical activity or lying flat for two hours after eating.
- Recommend that the patient not prepare his or her own food.

Intestinal Obstruction

- If oral intake is not contraindicated, encourage the patient to eat small meals of blenderized or strained foods that are low in fiber and residue. Offer the biggest meal early in the day. Many patients eat large portions of their favorite foods and then vomit. A gastric tube open to straight or intermittent drainage may relieve this need for frequent vomiting. With vomiting, foods high in potassium should be encouraged.
- In the case of "squashed stomach syndrome" have the patient eat frequent small meals, avoid nausea- and gas-producing foods, avoid high-fat or fried foods as well as foods that have strong odors. Limit fluid with meals, offering them 45 minutes before and after the meal.

Adapted from Gallagher-Allred, C. (1989). *Nutritional Care of the Terminally Ill* (pp. 151-195). Rockville, MD: Aspen Publishers, Inc.

ical treatments? or do they fall into the category of mandatory basic comfort care such as hygiene measures? Through use of the same decisional analysis that determines futility with other medical interventions (The Hastings Center, 1987), many have concluded that tube feeding and parenteral feeding are artificial methods of nutrition and therefore can be discontinued. Table 2 outlines considerations for examining the efficacy of foregoing aggressive nutrition support.

Prior to the 1970s, the technology of enteral and parenteral feedings was crude and often considered extraordinary or heroic care. Advanced technology, however, is now widely available both for institutional and home use. Some have argued that the availability of this technology compels an obligation to use it to feed. Others believe that the technology should be optional based on the individual's needs and circumstances. The American Dietetic Association (1992), American Medical Association (1986), and American Nurses Association (1988) have all published position papers asserting that health care personnel must comply with the patient's decision to forego medical treatment inclusive of nutrition and hydration.

Hence, it is—we emphasize—the patient's wish that is central to the decision to provide enteral or parenteral nutrition. The long term consistent viewpoint of the competent patient needs to be considered to help assure the authenticity of the decisions. If the patient has consistently stated a preference for or against interventions, an abrupt change of opinion necessitates a thorough review on the part of the health care team to safeguard the integrity of the patient. Bopp (1988) reminds the caregiver that a patient may be "incompetent to manage his affairs . . . but still competent to refuse to consent to medical treatment. Thus, the determination of competency depends upon the nature of the activity in question" (p. 33).

The alternatives regarding feeding options need to be clearly described to the patient. Lynn (1986) estimates that death will occur in a few days to two weeks without food or water. Both the risks and benefits of treatment and non-treatment must be clear. The patient's refusal of food and water needs to be concretely specified. It should not be an interpretation of a vague comment such as "Let me die . . ." or "Pull the plug . . . ." "In order that the

TABLE 2. Considerations for Examining the Efficacy of Forgoing or Discontinuing Aggressive Nutrition Support

I. Questions that can help to determine the potential burdens include:
    A. What is the level of risk for potential medical and metabolic complications from each available nutrition alternative?
    B. Will the administration of tube feeding or total parenteral nutrition at home or in a health care facility be contraindicted because of staffing, monitoring ability, or financial constraints?
    C. Will the nutritional benefits of the insertion of an enteral or parenteral feeding tube during hospitalization create feelings of abandonment if tube feeding is unavailable upon discharge?
II. Forgoing or discontinuing enteral or parenteral nutrition support may be considered when some or all of the following are present:
    A. Death is imminent, within hours or a few days.
    B. Enteral or parenteral feeding will probably worsen the condition, symptoms, or pain, such as during shock, when pulmonary edema or diarrhea, vomiting, or aspiration would cause further complications.
    C. A competent patient has expressed an informed preference not to receive aggressive nutrition support that would be ineffective in improving the quality of life and/or which may be perceived by the patient as undignified, degrading, and physically or emotionally unacceptable.
    D. If available and legally recognized, written advanced directives such as the "living will" or "durable power of attorney for medical care" may indicate the preference of an incompetent patient. Otherwise, the next of kin or patient appointed surrogate of an incompetent patient should be consulted about the patient's probable preference for the level of nutrition intervention, as well as state law.
III. Written ethical guidelines for assessing and implementing these considerations should be established through the facility's ethics committee, if available, and in accordance with legal guidance.
IV. Legal precedents and regulations or statutes establishing feeding parameters within local and state jurisdiction should be considered when deciding to require or forgo nutrition support. The facility's written protocol and legal counsel should also be consulted.

Reprinted with permission. American Dietetic Association (1992). "Position of the American Dietetic Association: Issues in Feeding the Terminally Ill Adult." *JADA* 92:996-1002.

fundamental right to life not be violated, a person who is deciding whether or not to refuse nutrition and hydration must be fully aware of the potential consequences, so that his choice is made 'voluntarily, knowingly and intelligently'" (Bopp, 1988, p. 38).

THE ECONOMICS OF FEEDING

It would be inappropriate and cost prohibitive to agencies and frequently detrimental to patients to require feeding and hydration for all who are dying. It would, on the other hand, be equally detrimental to withhold enteral or parenteral feeding from those for whom the feeding would improve the sense of well being, physically or symbolically. Each caregiver has an ethical and moral duty to conserve patients' health and life. Thus, we repeat, when there is doubt, feeding should be the rule.

The cost for enteral and parenteral feeding for the terminally ill adult is variable. The extent and duration of payment is based on the diagnosis and prognosis, the source of reimbursement, and the relationship of the feeding to survival. Health caregivers need to work with the interdisciplinary team and third party payers to maximize benefits for those who need enteral and parenteral feeding. Registered dietitians can provide expertise in determining the dimensions of value attached to diverse feeding issues.

CONCLUSION

The goals of palliative care should be approached from the physical, emotional, and spiritual needs and wishes of each individual patient. The extremes of patient nutrition-based fears range from being force fed to being neglected and/or abandoned. A basic fear is losing control of what happens to one's body. In that disease can be a powerfully humbling force, the patient can become dependent and fearful. One of the goals of hospice care is to ease or alleviate fear. The interdisciplinary health care team needs to reassure the patient, the family, and their friends that they can be trusted to respect the patient and his or her choices.

The registered dietitian has the skills to assess the nutritional status, the impact of disease processes, and the dietary patterns of the patient in order to develop an intervention plan that incorporates comfort needs, patient values, cost control, food safety, and optimal nutrition. The entire hospice team contributes to nutrition evaluation and counseling. The hospice dietitian's unique contribution to the work of the team is to optimize the nutrition component of care by continually updating and reinforcing applications drawn from nutrition science; by developing standards of care; and by giving advice on nutritional care, including potential drug-nutrient interactions. The services of a registered dietitian are integral to quality nutrition services for the hospice patient.

REFERENCES

American Dietetic Association. (1992). Position of the American Dietetic Association: Issues in feeding the terminally ill adult. *Journal of the American Dietetic Association, 92*: 996-1002.

American Medical Association. (1986). *Statement of the Council on Ethical and Judicial Affairs: Withholding or withdrawing life prolonging medical treatment.* Chicago: American Medical Association.

American Nurses Association. (1988). Guidelines on withdrawing or withholding food and fluids. *Ethics in nursing: Position statements and guidelines.* Kansas City, MO: American Nurses Association.

Bloch, A. (1990). *Nutrition and the cancer patient.* Rockville, MD: Aspen Publishers, Inc.

Bopp, J. (1988). Nutrition and hydration for patients: The constitutional aspects. *Issues in Law and Medicine, 4*(1), 3-52.

Gallagher-Allred, C. (1985). Dietitians are necessary in hospice programs. *The American Journal of Hospice Care, 2*(6), 11-12.

Gallagher-Allred, C. (1989). *Nutritional care of the terminally ill.* Rockville, MD: Aspen Publishers, Inc.

The Hastings Center. (1987). *Guidelines on the termination of life-sustaining treatment and the care of the dying.* Briarcliff Manor, NY.

Lynn, J. (1986). *By no extraordinary means.* Indiana, PA: Indiana University Press.

Mittleman, L. (1992). The legal implications of withholding and withdrawing nutrition support. *Support Line, XIV*(6), 1-6.

National Conference of Catholic Bishops' Committee. (1992, April 2). Nutrition and hydration: Moral and pastoral reflections. *Catholic News,* p. 18.

Caring for the Dying Child

Janice Miller-Thiel
Jacqueline J. Glover
Ev Beliveau

SUMMARY. In this paper we discuss the nutritional needs of terminally ill children. We delineate the physical, psychological, and developmental characteristics of children that differentiate them from adults *vis a vis* the nutritional aspects of their care. We highlight the special role of parents and suggest guidelines for dealing with the common nutritional needs of the dying child. We discuss ethical issues emphasizing the Baby Doe regulations, decision making for minors, and the benefits and burdens associated with permanently unconscious children.

INTRODUCTION

What do we do when a child no longer can or wants to eat? How do we continue to nurture, support, and care for the dying child

Janice Miller-Thiel, RN, is Assistant Director of Children's Hospice Services at the Children's Hospital of the Children's National Medical Center. Jacqueline J. Glover, PhD, is Director of the Program in Bioethics with Health Care Sciences at The George Washington University, and Philosopher in Residence at Children's National Medical Center. Ev Beliveau, RD, LD, is Senior Pediatric Clinical Dietitian at the Children's Hospital of the Children's National Medical Center.

Address correspondence to: Janice Miller-Thiel, RN, Children's Hospital of the Children's National Medical Center, 111 Michigan Avenue, NW, Washington, DC, 20010-2970.

[Haworth co-indexing entry note]: "Caring for the Dying Child." Miller-Thiel, Janice, Jacqueline J. Glover and Ev Beliveau. Co-published simultaneously in *The Hospice Journal* (The Haworth Press, Inc.) Vol. 9, Nos. 2/3, 1993, pp. 55-72; and: *Nutrition and Hydration in Hospice Care: Needs, Strategies, Ethics* (eds: Gallagher-Allred, Charlette, and Madalon O'Rawe Amenta) The Haworth Press, Inc., 1993, pp. 55-72. Multiple copies of this article/chapter may be purchased from The Haworth Document Delivery Center [1-800-3-HAWORTH; 9:00 a.m. - 5:00 p.m. (EST)].

© 1993 by The Haworth Press, Inc. All rights reserved.   *55*

whose nutritional needs are changing? At Children's Hospice Services of the Children's National Medical Center, Washington, DC we continually examine and evaluate these issues for families and professionals. The children we care for are in their own homes, either in the inner city of Washington, DC or the outlying suburbs of Maryland and Virginia. We meet with families from all walks of life. Some of the children have been ill since birth, others are only a few months into a life threatening illness. Sixty percent of the children we see have some form of cancer. The rest have cardiac and end-stage renal disease, various dystrophies, AIDS, cystic fibrosis and other genetic disorders and inborn errors of metabolism.

Hospice for children is an emerging field bringing with it few rules to help in feeding and hydration decision-making. Of the more than 1800 hospice organizations in the U.S., 500 admit children, and about 22 specialize in the care of terminally ill children. Of these 22, approximately eight are Medicare certified. Children's Hospice Services, part of Children's Hospital of the Children's National Medical Center, opened in 1981, was one of the first to become Medicare certified and JCAHO accredited. Despite this history and experience, we still do not have formulas; instead we find a case by case approach to be the most realistic. We work as a team utilizing an ethical framework to help ourselves and the families we serve.

Our priority is to help each child and his or her family determine how they want to live their remaining time together. Where do they see the most meaning? We then set up a plan to implement and support their decisions. As the body shuts down and the appetite decreases, parents can become quite desperate in their attempts to feed their child. Many parents tell stories of going to great lengths to prepare or purchase a requested food only to have the child take one look and refuse to eat it. This can lead to a battle of wills as the parent strives to assure food intake. At times like these the child's wishes are contrary to the parents' and the question can become who speaks for the child?

Characteristics of Children

Young children do not have sufficiently developed verbal skills or the ability to think abstractly. It is important that the hospice team be well versed in methods of eliciting communication from children. This can be done with drawings, play, age appropriate books, and one-on-one communication.

An important aspect of childhood development is magical thinking. Children believe they have the power to make something happen simply by thinking or wishing it so. Dying children may believe they will be cured through wishing and, therefore, think they do not need to eat to get better. The siblings of a dying child who have wished him or her harm may now find themselves feeling responsible for the illness and later the death. These siblings may lose their own appetites because of an overwhelming sense of guilt about their thoughts. The fear that they will be found out and be blamed keeps them in a constant state of apprehension. Communication with siblings, therefore, becomes important not only for their well being but also for that of the family.

All pertinent information about the particular disease the child has is given to siblings, as well as to the ill child and their parents. Rarely, however, do any of the adults involved ask questions that elicit the child's own view. The adults most often operate on the "official" view that has been given by the staff. Thus a question that we as caregivers ask all the children is, "How did you get sick?" The answers, always interesting, sometimes make us shake our heads and wonder where on earth they get their ideas. At other times their "logic" is apparent.

For example, a little girl told her nurse that she had cancer because she had gone outside without her mittens and hat the previous winter. She knew she had disobeyed her mother and was sure her cancer was the direct result. A sibling explained he hadn't had a thing to do with his brother's illness. His brother got sick from eating too much ice cream. We often comment among ourselves that children have their own math, and that for them 2 and 2 can make 6.

It is important to not assume that because a child is not asking questions that there are none, or that the situation is correctly understood. This is especially true in the nutritional domain. Often food is identified by a parent as the main "problem" but upon exploration with the child many other issues emerge. Children may use food to keep a parent at the bedside because they don't know how to say, "Don't go, I am afraid to be without you."

Children's observations about food can also be a signal to them of just how sick they are. Many children know that when they are well more limits are set on them and when they are sick or very sick they are given more latitude. When they see the extra effort in honoring special requests they often think they must be very sick. This can lead to further communication breakdown as they now have knowledge that they have not confirmed or discussed with anyone.

Hospice Nutrition Assessment and Education

Part of the role of the hospice team is to obtain an eating history that does not just focus on calories, weight, likes and dislikes, but also focuses on past eating behavior. This enables the team to sort through changes as they unfold.

Overall nutritional education and counseling need to take place from the very beginning. Education concerning ways to increase calories, understand nutritional needs, and recognize the changes the body is undergoing is essential to parental decision making. Parents need to have a sense that they have done all that can be done.

The counseling that helps them change from an active curative mode to an active palliative one without their focus becoming obsessive about food can be a challenge. If a fundamental obligation of a parent is to protect the child, many parents of terminally ill children feel they have failed and they often think that the last thing they can do for their child is to nurture and provide his or her favorite foods. Food may represent to them their one last effort to save the child. Parents need help in understanding that nutrition does not in all cases increase the body's ability to cure.

NUTRITIONAL MANAGEMENT OF TERMINALLY ILL CHILDREN

Adult versus Childhood Nutritional Characteristics

To meet the challenge that nutritional management and support for the terminally ill child poses, we must combine the professional caregivers' values to maximize the nutritional status with the family's values and practices in feeding their child. First we note the several significant differences between adults and children.

Children often do not have substantial subcutaneous fat stores to help them overcome the metabolic disturbances associated with malnutrition. In the child with cancer, for example, cachexia is triggered by the metabolic circuit that begins with increased tumor glycolysis that leads to increased gluconeogenesis and "Cori-cycling" in the liver, thus creating Protein Energy Malnutrition (PEM). The weight loss itself can cause weakness, lethargy, and depression. This syndrome of nutritional imbalances increases metabolic and caloric demands.

Secondly, in contrast to adults, usual nutritional support for children is aimed at promoting growth and development by achieving the nutritional recommendations identified in Table 1. Emphasis is

TABLE 1. Energy and Protein Requirements

Category	Age (years)	Reference Weight (kg)	REE[a] (cal/kg)	RDA (cal/kg)	Protein (gm/kg)
Infants	0.0-0.5	6	53	108	2.2
	0.5-1.0	9	56	98	1.6
Children	1-3	13	57	100	1.2
	4-6	20	47	90	1.1
	7-10	28	40	70	1.0
Males	11-14	45	32	55	1.0
	15-18	66	27	45	0.9
	19-24	72	25	40	0.8
Females	11-14	46	28	47	1.0
	15-18	55	25	40	0.8
	19-24	58	23	38	0.8

Adapted from *Recommended Dietary Allowances* (RDA) Tenth edition (1989) Food and Nutrition Board, National Academy of Sciences National Research Council
[a]REE—Resting energy expenditure computed from WHO equations

placed on nourishing the *growing* child. It is just this emphasis that parents and professionals must shift away from when the child is dying. Pediatric patients with PEM often have suboptimal growth and anthropometric indices (weight, height, weight for height, head circumference, tricep skin folds, mid arm muscle circumference) that both parents and caregivers are used to paying close attention to. Children with PEM are at higher risk for immune function abnormalities, muscle wasting, irritability, lethargy, and lack of interest in playing. All of these can exacerbate the clinical condition.

Thirdly, our society imposes moral values on parents who are made to feel ultimately responsible for their child's nutritional status. Suboptimal eating habits and poor nutritional health are often considered parental failures. "Did diet and nutrition cause my child's cancer?" they sometimes ask.

Illness and Children's Nutrition

This already complicated picture becomes even more complex when a chronic disease is added. Illness itself can lead to symptoms that interfere with a child's nutritional status.

Symptoms/patterns that might interfere with nutrition include:

• constipation, due to disease or high dose narcotics
• dry or sore mouth
• small bowel syndrome
• taste alterations
• nausea/vomiting
• food presented at times of day when appetite is lowest
• increased oral and respiratory secretions
• decreased tolerance for volume of foods.

If these symptoms are managed, caregivers may see an increase in appetite.

Psychological Concerns

Other major problems of reduced food intake are the related psychological concerns of the patient, family members, and professional caregivers. Parental involvement with nutrition is key. The parent/child interaction influences the child's food acceptance. Feeding children depends on more than just providing adequate, varied, and safe food.

Food is often the one thing parents and the child feel they can control. In hospice, the nutritional management focus changes as the child becomes more obviously terminally ill. The transition is difficult for all. Families often have become accustomed to the acute care setting in which emphasis is placed on maximizing nutritional management to enhance curative goals. In the acute care setting, there tends to be a sharper focus on assessment and management of the toxicities of treatment that may interfere with or affect nutritional status. Emphasis is placed on such things as the child's weight, caloric intake, fluid status, electrolyte balance, oral medications to correct nutrient deficiencies, and methods of caloric supplementation with the possible use of tube feedings.

Parents are constantly reminded of the importance of nutritional management to prevent or reverse PEM and its complications during the curative phase of treatment. They also strive to maximize their child's potential for growth, improved muscle function, overall performance, and feeling of well-being.

In the hospice setting all this is re-evaluated. As health care providers, we need to be sensitive to the child's clinical course in setting nutritional goals. These goals need to be measured and balanced to ensure that the benefit outweighs the burden for each individual family. This management is often complex and requires close coordination with a pediatric hospice interdisciplinary team of physicians, nurses, dietitians, social workers, and chaplains. Nutritional support is an important issue that must be addressed in the development of a comprehensive care plan.

With the dying child, one needs to balance baseline medical needs with the family's needs. Parents are the first to identify their child's change in status as she or he loses the ability or desire to eat or play. Some clearly do not want their last actions to be those of forcing their non-hungry child to eat or drink. They are comfortable in providing medications and enough liquid to keep their child's mouth and lips moist and comfortable. Perhaps they have witnessed the deaths of other family members and have seen the increased secretions, edema, abdominal discomfort, and pain that excess fluid in the system can produce. With that image in mind they may decide that artificial feedings are not for their dying child.

Many of these parents are surrounded by a family and social circle that support their view, but others may not be. Those that are not may need to look to the hospice to help explain and support their decisions to those who are challenging them. Hospice does not endorse any one decision as the right one. Rather it strives to determine what is best for a particular child at any given time.

Nutrition History

A child's nutrition history can provide the groundwork for effective nutrition counseling. Regardless of the child's prognosis, parents often focus on whether he or she is eating enough of the right foods according to long-established patterns. The dietitian is instrumental in offering individualized information to evaluate feeding options and nutritional strategies. General guidelines for feeding toddlers and children, and tips for overcoming some of the common nutrition problems that occur with terminal illness, are presented in Table 2. High calorie and high protein milk shake, and cookie and pudding recipes that parents and children can make at home appear in the Appendix.

"Questionable" Methods

The dietitian may face a particular challenge when the family uses self-prescribed special diets or questionable nutritional supplements in the belief that they have curative value. The goal is not to deny this choice to the family, but rather to educate them and help them seek a solution that will not be dangerous for the child.

Children with Problems Eating by Mouth

Critically and chronically ill children pose another nutritional challenge. Some children have never learned to eat. All their lives they have been fed through IV lines or tubes. This is often the case with children with multiple birth defects, nerve and muscle dysfunction, infantile spasms, and cardiac abnormalities. When oral feeding is contraindicated, it is important to provide non-nutritive stimulation. We may offer an infant a pacifier to suck during a nasal gastric feeding. Often we will hold the infant during the feeding just as if he or she were taking a bottle. They need this support.

Many of our critically ill children have had intensive care treatments and life support measures (respirators, feeding tubes, suctioning) which have imposed great stress to the mouth and throat. Their mouths are often sensitive and eating can be painful. Sometimes mastering these obstacles from the critical care period can extend into care at home. In the best of circumstances, these children can be slow in learning or relearning to eat.

There is a great deal to be said for inventiveness, enticement, and specially prepared foods. Children usually have their own motivations to eat. Often the key is gentle/non-demanding encouragement coupled with the extra step to make the food enticing (see Table 2). Undoubtedly the very sick child deserves consideration and respect for his or her choices as to whether or what to eat. It is important to not let food battles interfere with the family's time together.

ETHICAL ISSUES

As we move from curative to palliative treatment choices and as oral intake of food becomes difficult, the decisions of what is "extraordinary" and what is "ordinary" come into the foreground for active discussion and decision making. It is important to have an ethical framework to guide decisions, especially since they involve children, patients whom many consider unable to make "informed" choices.

Historical Influences

Despite the Cruzan decision supporting the permissibility of forgoing the medical provision of fluids and nutrition in adult medicine, concerns remain in pediatrics. There is a reluctance to forgo the medical provision of fluids and nutrition to infants and children that may stem from ambiguity in the so-called Baby Doe regula-

TABLE 2. Feeding Tips for Toddlers and Young Children

General Guidelines

Ensure a relaxed, calm, and positive approach during mealtime.

Allow adequate time for meals (30-45 minutes).

Minimize distractions during meal time (TV, computer games, toys).

Encourage normal family mealtimes/interactions/accompaniment with your child.

Serve small nutritious meals (4-6 meals vs. 3 traditional meals).

Help make every bite count. Top crackers, pretzels, other favorite snack foods with margarine, cheese, dips, peanut butter (even eaten from the spoon).

Offer non-traditional foods at different meal times. (Examples, have Breakfast at Dinner time. A pancake supper, with syrup on the side—dipping is fun! or have a nutritious dessert first!)

Use high calorie fruit juice and milk instead of water.

Add food coloring or flavored Kool-Aid to milk, for that little bit of pizzazz.

Read the labels on food containers to select the brand of ice cream, yogurt, and cheeses that are highest in calories. Offer your child his or her favorite toppings.

LOSS OF APPETITE

Take advantage of the times the child is awake and more interactive. Keep frozen foods around for convenient access to nutritious snacks and meals. Pre-portion and freeze the favorite leftovers.

Kids love color, shapes, and if feeling creative, like to help. (Perhaps take that mixing bowl to the bedside for your assistant's help.)

EARLY SATIETY

Offer smaller meals more frequently.

Limit the amount of liquids taken with meals.

Offer fluids with nutritional value.

DRY MOUTH

Dunk and dip foods into milk, juice, hot chocolate, sauces, dressings, or yogurt.

Offer juice popsicles (with polycose), or juice ice cubes, hard candy, or gum.

TABLE 2 (continued)

Offer foods with higher fluid content, such as cooked cereals, puddings, casseroles, canned sweetened fruits, or yogurt. Avoid extremely hot or cold foods.

ALTERED TASTE SENSATIONS

Offer foods at different temperatures.

Use flavorings to enhance and "Zip Up" the tastes, such as chocolate syrup, strawberry or vanilla.

Tart foods such as orange, lemon or grapefruit may be preferred.

Use seasonings such as parmesan cheese, mustard mixed with mayonnaise, lemon juice, onion, bacon.

SORE MOUTH

Avoid acidic or spicy foods and beverages (orange juice, pizza, spaghetti sauce, ketchup, lemonade, tomato). Use Kool-Aid, milk, or regular non-caffeinated soft drinks, instead.

Use soft, moist foods.

Use sauces, margarine, and gravies to mix food to desired consistency.

Make juice popsicles with banana slices; keep frozen pudding pops and ice cream bars on hand.

DIARRHEA

Try the BRAT diet (Bananas, Rice, Applesauce, and Toast). Drink liquids one hour after a meal instead of with a meal.

DIFFICULTY SWALLOWING

Provide small frequent meals of soft consistency (avoid "thin" liquids) add butter, margarine, sour cream or cream cheese to liquify foods.

tions, now incorporated into the federal Child Abuse Amendments of 1984 (Department of Health and Human Services, 1985). The regulations specify that as a condition of receiving state grants under the Child Abuse Prevention and Treatment Act (Public Law, 1974), states must establish programs and/or procedures within the state's child protective service system to respond to reports of medical neglect, including reports of the withholding of medically indicated treatment for disabled infants with life-threatening conditions. According to the regulations:

The term 'withholding of medically indicated treatment' means the failure to respond to the infant's life-threatening conditions by providing treatment (including appropriate nutrition, hydration, and medication) which, in the treating physician's (or physicians') reasonable medical judgment, will be most likely to be effective in ameliorating or correcting all such conditions, except that the term does not include the failure to provide treatment (other than appropriate nutrition, hydration, or medication) to an infant when, in the treating physician's (or physicians') reasonable medical judgment any of the following circumstances apply: (i) The infant is chronically and irreversibly comatose; (ii) The provision of such treatment would merely prolong dying, not be effective in ameliorating or correcting all of the infant's life-threatening conditions, or otherwise be futile in terms of the survival of the infant; or (iii) The provision of such treatment would be virtually futile in terms of the survival of the infant and the treatment itself under such conditions would be inhumane. (p. 14888)

Interpretation of the regulations depends on the meaning inferred by the term 'appropriate.' Those who would argue that it is always appropriate would interpret the regulations to require the medical provision of fluids and nutrition. Those who would argue that the medical provision of fluids and nutrition may be ethically withheld or withdrawn would interpret the regulations to permit this in appropriate circumstances (Paris & Fletcher, 1987). Considered legal judgment seems to favor the latter interpretation in light of the Cruzan decision (Barnett, 1990).

All would agree that the Baby Doe regulations reflect an underlying concern for protecting the interests of vulnerable patients. The decisions we make on behalf of others require more scrutiny than those we make for ourselves. Unlike the Cruzan case where the Missouri court ultimately decided there was clear and convincing evidence of the adult Nancy's wishes, decisions on behalf of critically ill infants and children cannot be based on the values of the particular patient. As parents and professional caregivers, we struggle to articulate the shared values that should inform these decisions.

Decision Making for Children

Whose Responsibility?

Who is the appropriate spokesperson for the child? Obviously the presumption goes to the parents. We believe that their strong bonds of affection and commitment will most likely yield the greatest concern for the well-being of the child. It is the primary responsibility of parents to protect children and to provide the best decisions and support possible for their welfare. The interests of parents and their children are inextricably linked. Harm to a child also constitutes harm to the mother or father. The family relationship, itself, is a given value for both parents and children, and society limits interference into this private realm. Additionally, it is the parents who bear the responsibility for the life-long consequences of decisions.

But professional caregivers also share responsibility for decisions. Parents and professionals must work together in a therapeutic alliance on behalf of the child. Neither is the mere instrument of the other's preferences. Just as parents cannot act as surrogate health care professionals, professionals cannot act as surrogate parents. Both perspectives are necessary.

Maturity Level of the Child

Additionally, mature children should be involved in decisions about their own care to the extent possible. Siblings, likewise, should be included and have the truth shared with them. For example, the child's ability to understand cause and effect will have a large impact on what is perceived as a burden. What could be a burden for a four year old might not be for a 12 year old. The four year old only knows that the tube hurts being inserted and that it feels uncomfortable while it is in. She or he has no sense of what it has to do with his or her stomach and how it feels. What he or she does know is that it feels better when the tube is out and will be most helpful in removing it.

Consideration of the benefit and burden is very different for the 12 year old who may see the correlation between the discomfort with the tube and the comfort of getting medications through it or enough fluids to keep his or her mouth moist. The patient, family, and professional caregivers all contribute important information about the appropriate goals of therapy and their associated benefits and burdens.

When There Is Conflict

Sometimes, however, there is conflict. Children are not only members of their immediate families, but also of the broader community. Community concern may justify the protection of individuals from the harms inflicted by their families. As a society, we look to health care professionals to help determine when family members are not acting in the best interests of their children. The assessment of when community standards of best interest ought to outweigh a family determination is extremely difficult. There is a strong presumption favoring life. But when life cannot be preserved or the chance of survival is minimal, burdens such as repeated pain and suffering from invasive procedures, fear, immobilization, prolonged hospitalization, and isolation from family and friends, must be considered.

In dealing with such disagreements strategies for resolution include: (a) obtaining the most current, factual information regarding points of controversy; (b) reaching consensus about the meaning of key terms (like extraordinary and ordinary); (c) agreeing on a common framework of moral principles to guide discussions; and (d) engaging in a balanced discussion of the positive and negative aspects of a particular viewpoint. Patient care conferences or institutional ethics committees can serve as useful forums (Rushton & Glover, 1990).

It is expected that discussion about ethical issues will be highly emotional. This is particularly true when we are talking about fluids and nutrition. Who can forget the powerful images of the original Baby Doe, who was not fed because of the decision to forgo correctional surgery for duodenal atresia? The case highlights our instinct to nurture and not abandon the young. Some would argue that the value of helping, or at least not harming, always requires the provision of fluids and nutrition.

Such an argument depends on the assumption that the provision of fluids and nutrition is always beneficial. Some would deny that fluids and nutrition are medical treatments, but rather basic care like hygiene. Yet even if it is assumed that such care is not medical, if it causes discomfort or suffering, it is difficult to see how it can be viewed as an act of caring.

We compound the dilemma when our choice of language is powerful and possibly misleading, as in the use of words like starvation. We may confuse the situation by using such powerful language in cases in which the child cannot or does not experience hunger or thirst. To ignore the reality of his or her experience is to risk greater burdens for the child. To base the moral argument about fluids and nutrition on their unique nature is to risk ignoring good patient-centered care. At the heart of the moral consideration of the use of fluids and nutrition is the best interest of the child, which must be based on an assessment of the total benefits and burdens involved.

In addition to concerns about not harming children by failing to provide adequate fluids and nutrition, caregivers are also concerned about their role in the child's death. Many are particularly uncomfortable when the medical provision of fluids and nutrition is the only life-sustaining therapy, as is often the case with the permanently unconscious. Other technologies, like ventilators, seem different. A child who is taken off the ventilator still has the air to breathe if he or she is able. A child cannot possibly survive without other persons supplying adequate fluids and nutrition.

Yet are these cases really so different? We would consider the cause of death to be brain damage secondary to anoxia for the child from whom the ventilator is withdrawn because of his or her inability to breathe without medical assistance. Wouldn't the same anoxia be the cause of death for the child who has lost the ability to eat or drink? Aren't we also sure that a child will die when we discontinue dialysis? Rather than cause of death or certainty of death, the moral argument must revolve around an assessment of burdens and benefits.

Benefits and Burdens in Permanently Unconscious Children

How does one assess benefits and burdens in a permanently unconscious child? In such a state, a child is not capable of experiencing any of the things we usually consider as benefits or burdens. Except for continued basic biological maintenance, it is difficult to say how we are benefitting the child at all. The child cannot interact with his or her family or experience any other pleasures and satisfactions associated with daily life. Yet the child is not being burdened since he or she cannot experience pain or suffering. Lacking any interest in enhancing benefits or reducing burdens, a best interests standard would not appear to apply.

The Relational Potential Standard

Some would propose the addition of a relational potential standard addressing the lack of ability to interact with the environment (McCormick, 1974). In such cases life-sustaining treatment may be withheld or withdrawn. Rather than assume that any interests must be served when there are no corresponding burdens, many would argue that treatment may be limited or withdrawn if most of the reasons for that treatment are missing—better function, fewer symptoms, the opportunity for human relationships, or greater opportunity to achieve life's goals. Whether treatment is forgone or not will depend heavily on the values of the family (President's Commission, 1983).

Although the relational potential standard is clearly followed in adults, as evidenced by the Cruzan case, and is mentioned in the Baby Doe regulations, fluids and nutrition are rarely withheld in permanently unconscious children. This may be due partly to difficulties in diagnosis (Ashwal et al., 1992). Mostly, however, it is probably due to our attitudes toward children generally and our particularly strong desire to nurture them. Additionally, infants do not look physically as unnatural as adults when they are permanently unconscious (Miraie & Mahowald, 1988). Such attitudes are changing, especially as we struggle to give children the same consideration we give to adults. We are now asking ourselves, "Is the prolongation of the unconscious life of a child an act of caring?"

CONCLUSION

In the case of children, the presumption still remains strong in favor of providing fluids and nutrition. Although they may be justifiably withheld or withdrawn when the burdens outweigh the benefits or when there is no relational potential, we must still be concerned about the slippery slope. One author has called the withdrawal of fluids and nutrition "the non-treatment of choice" for the "biologically tenacious" (Callahan, 1983). We should be extremely careful when we are talking about chronically ill children who must be fed through medical means, but otherwise can lead very active lives. Our challenge is to acknowledge the special character of fluids and nutrition without losing sight of the child and family for whom we are caring.

REFERENCES

Ashwal, S., Bale, J. F. Jr., Coulter, D. L., Eiben, R., Garg, B. P., Hill, A., Myer, E. C., Nordgren, R. E., Sheumon, D. A., Sunder, T. R., & Walker, R. W. (1992). The persistent vegetative state in children: Report of The Child Neurology Society Ethics Committee. *Annals of Neurology, 32*(40), 570-576.

Barnett, T. (1990). Baby Doe: Nothing to fear but fear itself. *Journal of Perinatology, 10*(3), 307-311.

Callahan, D. (1983). Feeding the dying. *Hastings Center Report, 13*(22).

Department of Health and Human Services. (1985). *Federal Register, 50*(72) (45 CFR Part 1340).

McCormick, R. (1974). To save or let die: The dilemma of modern medicine. *Journal of the American Medical Association, 229*(172).

Miraie, E.D., & Mahowald, M.B. (1988). Withholding nutrition from seriously ill newborn infants: A parent's perspective. *The Journal of Pediatrics, 113*(2), 262-265.

Paris, J.J., & Fletcher, A.B. (1987). Withholding of nutrition and fluids in the hopelessly ill patient. *Ethical and Legal Issues in Perinatology, 14*(2), 367-377.

Presidents Commission for the Study of Ethical Problems in Medicine and Biomedical and Behavioral Research. (1983). *Deciding to Forego Life-Sustaining Treatment*, p. 171-196. U.S. Government Printing Office, Washington, DC

Public Law, § 92-247, 42 U.S.C. § 5101, et seg. (1974).

Rushton, C.H., & Glover, J.J. (1990). Involving parents in decisions to forego life-sustaining treatment for critically ill infants and children. *Clinical Issues in Critical Care Nursing, 1*(1), 206-214.

APPENDIX

SUGGESTED RECIPES FOR HIGH CALORIE/HIGH PROTEIN FOODS FOR CHILREN

SUPER SHAKE

> 1 cup ice cream
> 1 cup milk
> 1 package instant breakfast powder

Mix well. Total calories: 560 per recipe. (Varies with instant breakfast flavor and fat percent of ice cream.)

PEANUT BUTTER LOGS

> 1 cup dry milk powder
> 1/2 lb peanut butter
> 1/2 cup honey**
> 1 cup Rice Krispies cereal
> 1 cup Bran Flakes cereal
> 1/2 cup raisins

Mix all ingredients well. Flatten mixture into a 13×9×2 inch pan. Chill overnight. Cut into 2"×1" logs.
Total calories: 160 per log.

SUPER PUDDING

> 2 cups milk
> 2 tablespoons vegetable oil
> 1 package (4 1/2 ounces) instant pudding mix
> 3/4 cup dry milk powder

Stir milk and oil; add instant pudding and mix well. Pour 1/2 cup servings into dishes.
Total calories: 200 per 1/2 cup serving.

**NOTE: Do not give honey to children less than one year old.

Appetite Stimulants in Terminal Care: Treatment of Anorexia

Phyllis A. Grauer

SUMMARY. Anorexia is a common problem in terminally ill patients. The loss of appetite brings with it physical, psychological, and social problems. Effective treatment, therefore, should be multidimensional. The pharmacist is well-positioned to evaluate the appropriate use of medications for their effects on appetite, weight gain, mood, nausea, and anorexia. Studies have demonstrated that megestrol acetate has the most positive results in patients with advanced cancer and human immunodeficiency virus. Other medications studied have a less significant impact. Total parenteral nutrition can also sustain meaningful life for many terminally ill patients, but it is rarely successful in alleviating the anorexia associated with terminal illness.

INTRODUCTION

The physical effects of weight loss that lead to cachexia and the decreased energy associated with anorexia can be distressing to the

Phyllis A. Grauer, RPh, is Clinical Pharmacist for Hospice at Riverside, Columbus, OH.

Address correspondence to: Phyllis A. Grauer, Hospice at Riverside, 3595 Olentangy River Rd., Columbus, OH, 43214.

The author wishes to thank Mellar P. Davis, MD, for his support and contribution to this article.

[Haworth co-indexing entry note]: "Appetite Stimulants in Terminal Care: Treatment of Anorexia." Grauer, Phyllis A. Co-published simultaneously in *The Hospice Journal* (The Haworth Press, Inc.) Vol. 9, Nos. 2/3, 1993, pp. 73-83: and: *Nutrition and Hydration in Hospice Care: Needs, Strategies, Ethics* (eds: Gallagher-Allred, Charlette, and Madalon O'Rawe Amenta) The Haworth Press, Inc., 1993, pp. 73-83. Multiple copies of this article/chapter may be purchased from The Haworth Document Delivery Center [1-800-3-HAWORTH; 9:00 a.m. - 5:00 p.m. (EST)].

© 1993 by The Haworth Press, Inc. All rights reserved.

patient, the caregiver, and/or the health care provider. Reports indicate that up to 87% of terminally ill patients experience anorexia (Bruera, 1992). Should anorexia be treated and if so when? When considering the options of using medication to stimulate appetite or of providing supplemental nutrition, it is essential to evaluate if these interventions will genuinely improve the quality of the patient's life or extend his or her meaningful time.

Decisions regarding nutritional support of the terminally ill should be dealt with in the same manner in which all quality of life issues are addressed. The patient and family have the right to be given complete and accurate information about the options available to them. This knowledge gives them the power to remain in control of their lives by making educated decisions about their treatment. Since rational decisions are best made when the patient is not in a state of crisis, dialogue should begin early in the course of the disease.

ETIOLOGY OF ANOREXIA AND CACHEXIA

In order to choose the appropriate therapy for anorexia and cachexia, it is necessary to review their causes. Researchers have focused predominantly on anorexia and cachexia in patients terminally ill with either cancer or human immunodeficiency virus (HIV) infections.

The causes of anorexia and cachexia in cancer patients are many. Systemic effects of a malignant disease can suppress appetite centrally and increase basal metabolic rate thus leading to weight loss. Altered substrate utilization leading to protein catabolism occurs through the Cori cycle. Increased levels of endogenous peptides such as glucagon, insulin, cholecystokinin, and calcitonin can inhibit food intake. Satietins, a family of alpha-1-glycoproteins, have potent and selective anorectic activities. The presence of tumor can trigger the immune system to release cytokines. Interleukin-1, tumor necrosis factor, and interferon-alpha have been specifically linked with anorexia (Bruera, 1992).

Anorexia

Anorexia is one of the leading culprits in body wasting that is a major problem in patients with HIV-associated cachexia. Other factors include malabsorption, altered metabolism of nutrients, chronic diarrhea, and coincidental opportunistic infections and their treatments.

Nausea

One obvious cause of anorexia is nausea. Sixty eight percent of patients with advanced cancer have chronic nausea, which is sometimes accompanied by intractable vomiting (Bruera, 1992). There are several factors directly associated with malignancy that may cause nausea. One is the bowel obstruction that often accompanies ovarian and colorectal cancers. "Squashed-stomach syndrome" can result from hepatomegaly or extensive tumor involvement in the peritoneal cavity. Paralytic ileus may accompany peritoneal implants of carcinoma. Both endogenous and exogenous substances circulating in the blood can activate the chemoreceptor trigger zone thus stimulating the vomiting center.

Certain advanced malignancies produce hypercalcemia which can result in anorexia and nausea. Increased intracranial pressure from brain metastases can cause nausea and vomiting as well as headache and changes in mental status. Nausea and vomiting associated with movement may develop when disease or medication affects the vestibular apparatus (Storey, 1991). Nausea is seen in patients with hepatic and renal failure from hyperbilirubinemia and uremia respectively. In addition, chemotherapy, radiation therapy, or high dose narcotics are also major offenders.

Many of these causes of nausea can be treated effectively with medications. Since nausea is a major cause of anorexia, it is imperative that chronic nausea be treated before attempting to implement additional treatment of anorexia.

TREATMENT OF ANOREXIA AND CACHEXIA

Anorexia and resulting malabsorption can be effectively ameliorated by therapies ranging from minor dietary modification to invasive feeding modalities such as total parenteral nutrition (TPN). In choosing a therapy for the terminally ill patient, emphasis should be placed on simplicity of administration, efficacy, and cost. Patient and caregiver should be allowed to focus on enjoying quality time rather than having to deal with high technology interventions that can be expensive, cumbersome, and uncomfortable (Loprinzi, Ellison, Goldberg, Michalak, & Burch, 1990).

Simple Dietary Therapies

Simple dietary adjustments can render food more appealing to the anorectic patient. Dietitians have a range of suggestions to improve appetite and increase caloric intake. One might be a cocktail or a glass of red wine before a meal to help stimulate appetite. Often with the help of the dietitian, the family can easily adapt ordinary foods to maximize benefit. Commercially available nutritional supplements may also be useful.

Total Parenteral Nutrition

A case can be made for limited use of total parenteral nutrition (TPN) in terminal care. When patients are in the early stages of the terminal phase of their disease, they are often able to lead full and active lives. TPN may be appropriate if patients are unable to ingest enough calories to sustain their activity level due to a non-functioning gastrointestinal tract (Fainsinger, Chan, & Bruera, 1992). An inoperable bowel obstruction or short bowel syndrome are two examples of such medical situations.

In general, however, TPN is not an effective treatment for the anorexia associated with encroaching terminal illness. The placement of a central line can induce a pneumothorax and can also lead to catheter related sepsis. As the patient's physical condition declines, organ failure frequently sets in. Under these conditions TPN can result in electrolyte imbalance and fluid accumulation, and it can complicate the management of renal failure or congestive heart failure. Patients and families who request questionable intravenous feedings such as TPN will often reconsider when the potential dangers are explained to them.

Pharmacological Interventions

The pharmacological approach to appetite stimulation is gaining popularity. Research has identified medications that stimulate appetite, increase weight gain, and improve the patient's sense of well being. A review of some of these findings follows.

Cyproheptadine (Periactin®)

Cyproheptadine, an antihistamine with antiseratonergic properties, has been anecdotally reported to benefit cancer patients. Kardinal et al. (1990) conducted a randomized controlled clinical trial in patients with advanced malignancies who received either 8 mg of cyproheptadine orally three times a day or placebo. Although this study demonstrated that the drug stimulated appetite mildly, compared to placebo it did not enhance weight gain.

Hydrazine Sulfate

Hydrazine sulfate in doses of 60 mg three times a day has been shown to stimulate appetite and promote or stabilize weight in patients with advanced cancer. This phosphoenolpyruvate carboxykinase inhibitor used in commercial manufacturing processes decreases amino acid flux, improves serum albumin levels, and controls glucose intolerance in humans. Reported side effects have been mild to moderate lightheadedness and nausea (Nelson & Walsh, 1991). There is conflicting data about its benefit in lung cancer patients.

Corticosteroids

Dexamethasone. The potent glucocorticoid corticosteroid, dexamethasone, when given orally in doses of 0.75 mg and 1.5 mg four times a day to patients with preterminal gastrointestinal cancer was well tolerated and caused no specific toxicities (Moertel, Schutte, Reitemeier, & Hahn, 1974). Although it initially significantly increased appetite, it did not favorably affect either weight gain or survival in patients with far advanced malignant disease.

Oral Methylprednisolone. In order to evaluate its effect on pain control, psychiatric status, appetite, nutritional status, daily activity, and performance, oral methylprednisolone was compared to placebo in a 14 day, randomized, double-blind crossover study of 40 terminally ill cancer patients (Bruera, Roca, Cedaro, Carrar, & Charon, 1985). The patients received doses of 16 mg orally twice a day. Compared to controls, pain intensity decreased in the study patients. Appetite and food consumption were significantly improved but nutritional status remained unchanged. Side effects of treatment were anxiety, fluid retention, and a Cushingoid appearance occurring in approximately 5% of the patients.

Prednisone. O'Shaughnessy (1989) reported on doses of 5 mg to 50 mg of prednisone, a corticosteroid with combined glucocorticoid and mineralocorticoid action, given orally twice a day for appetite stimulation. Generally, the need for dose escalation of this drug increases as the patient's prognosis worsens. In order to take advantage of its peak appetite stimulating effect, the best time to administer prednisone is four hours prior to meals. One advantage of prednisone over the pure glucocorticoid drugs such as dexamethasone is its decreased potential for Cushingoid changes. Prednisone also appears to produce an improvement in a patient's sense of well-being.

Megestrol Acetate (Megace®)

Multiple trials with megestrol acetate, a synthetic orally active progestational agent used in the treatment of breast and endometrial carcinomas, have demonstrated substantial improvement in appetite and food consumption in cancer and AIDS patients. In one study of patients receiving 800 mg of megestrol a day, an average weight gain of 14.2 lbs (6.5 kg) was reported. These changes in body weight were not attributed to fluid retention but appeared to be predominately fat. Studies of doses ranging from 160 mg to 1600 mg a day have generally concluded that greater weight gain occurs with higher doses. Long term use of megestrol appears to be safe in doses up to 800 mg a day (Mahayni & Minor, 1991). Although the mechanism of action of megestrol acetate in anorexia is unknown, evidence suggests that it may inhibit tumor necrosis factor (Mahayni & Minor, 1991; Bruera, Macmillan, Kuehn, Hanson, & Mac-Donald, 1990).

Patients receiving megestrol had fewer complaints of nausea and vomiting than those receiving placebo (Tchekmedyian et al., 1992). In addition, those patients who had lost a taste for food or had an aversion to sweets showed improvement while taking megestrol. Overall, megestrol acetate is well tolerated. The side effects appear to be mild; dyspnea (6%), edema (10-16%), hyperglycemia (2%), deep vein thrombosis (4%).

Certainly a major disadvantage of megestrol acetate for appetite stimulation is the cost. The largest dose currently available is a 40 mg tablet, hence it would take 20 tablets a day to complete an 800 mg dose. Not only might patient acceptance and compliance be problems but cost might be prohibitive, as well. For information about costs of medications commonly used as appetite stimulants, see Table 1.

The results of these clinical trials are promising, yet more research is needed to determine the optimal dose and the benefit of megestrol in the anorectic terminally ill patients.

Dronabinol (Marinol®)

Dronabinol, a commercially available preparation of delta-9-tetrahydrocannabinol in sesame oil, may be helpful in the alleviation of the chronic refractory nausea and vomiting associated with anorexia. Ongoing studies are evaluating the effectiveness of dronabinol as an appetite stimulant in HIV patients (Conant, Roy, Shepard, & Plasse, 1991). Preliminary results have failed to show significant weight gain; however, improvement in both appetite and mood have been noted.

One study tested various dosages. Dronabinol doses of 2.5 mg twice a day up to 5 mg three times a day appeared to be effective, but 2.5 mg once a day showed no results. Adverse effects included dizziness, fluid retention, somnolence, and dissociation. Although study doses were given one hour prior to meals, it has been noted that patients experienced fewer adverse effects if the dose is given one hour after breakfast and lunch. This is particularly true with elderly patients who are more sensitive to the drug than younger adults (Nelson & Walsh, 1991).

TABLE 1. Costs of Medications Commonly Used for Appetite Stimulation

Medication	Dose	Approximate Cost per Day*
Cyproheptadine		
Periactin®	8 mg three times a day.	$ 2.15
Generic	(2 × 4 mg tablets/dose)	$ .25
Dexamethasone		
Decadron®	.75-1.5 mg@ four times	$ 2.00
Generic	a day.	$ .60
Methylprednisolone		
Medrol®	16 mg twice a day.	$ 2.25
Generic		$ 1.60
Prednisone		
Deltasone®	5-50 mg@ twice a day.	$ .30
Generic		$ .50
Megestrol Acetate	160-800 mg@ a day in	
Megace®	divided doses.	$19.65
Generic	(20 × 40 mg tablets/day@)	$15.00
Dronabinol	2.5 mg twice to 5 mg	
Marinol®	three times a day.	$13.15

*Wholesale prices are based on 1991-1992 Blue Book Average Wholesale Price, First Databank Annual Directory of Pharmaceuticals, The Hearst Corp. @Maximum dose used for determining cost per day.

Symptom Management

Pain Control

Many symptoms that are common in terminally ill patients, if left untreated, can lead to anorexia. It is essential that pain be adequately treated. Analgesics should be administered so that the patient is pain free yet not too drowsy to be able to eat.

Narcotic analgesics, the mainstay of chronic cancer pain management, unfortunately have side effects that can lead to anorexia, nausea, and vomiting. Although these side effects are generally transient, providing the patient with an anti-emetic agent for use as needed can prevent them from becoming a problem. Constipation, which is always anticipated with the use of narcotic analgesics, should be treated prophylactically.

Gastric Motility

Gastroparesis, sometimes caused by narcotic analgesics, often occurs in terminally ill patients. Metoclopramide (Reglan®) 10 mg to 20 mg before meals and at bedtime can increase gastric motility thus preventing anorexia due to gastric fullness. Although effective in patients with partial obstruction or constipation, it is contraindicated in complete bowel obstruction.

Depression

Depression in terminal illness can also contribute to anorexia. Psychological intervention is fundamental; and medications are appropriate adjuncts. Tricyclic antidepressants have the added benefit of appetite stimulation. Antidepressants that are known to decrease appetite such as fluoxetine (Prozac®) should be avoided. Any other medications, including some antidepressants, that have been associated with taste disturbances leading to anorexia should also be avoided.

Histamine$_2$-antagonists are useful in patients who have anorexia due to hypersecretion of gastric fluids. Drugs such as ranitidine (Zantac®), famotidine (Pepcid®), and cimetidine (Tagamet®) often are effective when given as one time doses at bedtime.

Mouth Care

Mouth care is important in maintaining a good appetite. Teeth should be brushed regularly and dentures kept clean. A dentist should be consulted for dentures with altered fit due to weight loss or tooth and gum problems. Aggressive treatment of mouth sores can facilitate eating. Normal saline mouth rinses are helpful for irritated mucosal membranes. Commercially available mouthwashes may be beneficial, however, the solutions that contain alcohol can irritate inflamed oral tissues. If the patient develops a candida infection, nystatin swish, ketoconazole tablets, or other antifungal agents should be used. Herpes simplex can be treated with oral acyclovir. Lidocaine viscous is one of many topical preparations that can be used at mealtime to anesthetize painful areas. Combinations of viscous lidocaine, diphenhydramine, and Maalox® or sucralfate slurries relieve chemotherapy induced stomatitis.

CONCLUSION

Anorexia is a prevalent problem in terminally ill patients. There are many interventions that can help alleviate the problems associated with the loss of appetite and weight loss. Because of the multidimensional issues surrounding anorexia, utilization of the expertise of all hospice team members is needed to most effectively address this symptom.

Reversible factors contributing to anorexia should be identified and treated. Enlisting the assistance of a pharmacist will provide the team with valuable assistance for appropriate pharmacological interventions. Medications that can potentially suppress appetite should be avoided if possible. Medication dosage schedules should be adjusted so that patients do not take so many medications at mealtimes that they essentially fill up on pills. The pharmacist with the dietitian, nurse, physician, and patient and family can evaluate the appropriateness of using medication to stimulate appetite. Megestrol acetate clearly has the most promising benefit on appetite and weight gain, however, cost and patient compliance are limiting factors. Other drugs such as corticosteroids and dronabinol may be employed if pain and nausea are also symptoms.

It is important for practitioners not to offer therapeutic interventions to satisfy their own need to fix the problem of anorexia. Patient, family, and hospice team should decide which, if any, treatment is appropriate to enhance quality of life.

REFERENCES

Bruera, E., Macmillan, K., Kuen, N., Hanson, J., & MacDonald, R.N. (1990). A controlled trial of megestrol acetate on appetite, caloric intake, nutritional status, and other symptoms in patients with advanced cancer. *Cancer, 66*, 1279-1282.

Bruera, E., Roca, E., Cedaro, L., Carrar, S., & Charon, R. (1985). Action of oral methylprednisolone in terminal cancer patients: A prospective randomized double-blind study. *Cancer Treatment Reports, 9* (7-8), 751-754.

Bruera, E. (1992). Current pharmacological management of anorexia in cancer patients. *Oncology, 6* (1), 125-130.

Conant, M., Roy, D., Shepard, K.V., & Plasse, T.F. (1991, March). Dronabinol enhances appetite and controls weight loss in HIV patients. *Proceedings of ASCO, 10*, 34.

Fainsinger, R.L., Chan, K., & Bruera, E. (1992). Total parenteral nutrition for a terminally ill patient? *Journal of Palliative Care, 8*(2), 30-32.

Kardinal, C.G., Loprinzi, C.L., Schaid, D.J., Hass, A.C., Dose, A.M., Athman, L., Maillirad, J.A., McCormack, G.W., Gerstner, J.B., & Schray, M.F. (1990). A controlled trial of cyproheptadine in cancer patients with anorexia and/or cachexia. *Cancer, 65*, 2657-2662.

Loprinzi, C., Ellison, N., Goldberg, R.M., Michalak, J.C., & Burch, P.A. (1990). Alleviation of cancer anorexia and cachexia: Studies of the Mayo clinic and the North Central Cancer Treatment Group. *Seminars in Oncology, 17*(6) (Suppl. 9), 8-12.

Mahayni, H., & Minor, J. (1991). Megestrol acetate in AIDS-related cachexia. *American Journal of Hospital Pharmacy, 48*(11), 2479-2480.

Moertel, C., Schutte, A., Reitemeier, R.J., & Hahn, R.G. (1974). Corticosteroid therapy of preterminal gastrointestinal cancer. *Cancer, 33*, 1607-1609.

Nelson, K., & Walsh, D. (1991). Management of anorexia cachexia syndrome. *The Cancer Bulletin, 3*(5), 403-405.

O'Shaughnessy, C.O. (1989). *Hospice medicine–Pain control in advanced cancer.* Detroit, MI: Charles Owen O'Shaughnessy, MD.

Storey, P. (1991). Medical management of nonchemotherapy-induced nausea and vomiting in advanced cancer patients. *The Cancer Bulletin, 43*(5), 433-436.

Tchekmedyian, N.S., Hickman, M., Siau, J., Greco, F.A., Keller, J., Browder, H., & Aisner, J. (1992). Megestrol acetate in cancer anorexia and weight loss. *Cancer, 69*(5), 1268-1274.

Maximizing Foodservice
in an Inpatient Hospice Setting

Kathleen Drew Kidd

Mary Pat Lane

SUMMARY. The philosophy of maximizing patient comfort and enhancing quality of life impacts on all aspects of foodservice in an inpatient hospice setting. The foodservice department's focus in the palliative care environment is to meet patients' physical, psychological, and social needs. The menu incorporates variety and comfort foods to meet the special requests of hospice patients. Food production and delivery provides for flexibility in meal preferences and meal serving times. Finally, sanitation standards and inservice training extend beyond the main foodservice operation to include the hospice "family" kitchen to protect the hospice patient from foodborne infections.

INTRODUCTION

Patient comfort is a primary tenet of palliative care philosophy and an important consideration when planning and providing nutri-

---

Kathleen Drew Kidd, MS, RD, LD, is Director, Nutrition and Food Services, of the Washington Hospice, a program of The Washington Home, Washington, DC. Mary Pat Lane, MS, RD, is Food and Nutrition Services Manager of Hospice of Northern Virginia, Arlington, VA.

Address correspondence to: Kathleen Drew Kidd, 17012 MacDuff Ave., Olney, MD 20835.

The authors offer special thanks to Clemmie Saxton, PhD, RD, Howard University Department of Nutrition Services, Washington, DC; Paul Araujo, RD, Stella Maris Hospice, Baltimore, MD; and the staffs of our own hospices.

[Haworth co-indexing entry note]: "Maximizing Foodservice in an Inpatient Hospice Setting." Kidd, Kathleen Drew and Mary Pat Lane. Co-published simultaneously in *The Hospice Journal* (The Haworth Press, Inc.) Vol. 9, Nos. 2/3, 1993, pp. 85-106: and: *Nutrition and Hydration in Hospice Care: Needs, Strategies, Ethics* (eds: Gallagher-Allred, Charlette, and Madalon O'Rawe Amenta) The Haworth Press, Inc., 1993, pp. 85-106. Multiple copies of this article/chapter may be purchased from The Haworth Document Delivery Center [1-800-3-HAWORTH; 9:00 a.m. - 5:00 p.m. (EST)].

© 1993 by The Haworth Press, Inc. All rights reserved.

tious food in the hospice. The goal is that this comfort will allow the patient to control his or her remaining life in a meaningful way (Amenta & Bohnet, 1986). Planning and supplying appealing, enjoyable, nutritious food for seriously ill patients with compromised appetites and eating capacities is the challenge of the foodservice department, which also strives to maximize the comfort of patient and family through the medium of food choice. In these ways, the foodservice department becomes an integral component in enhancing the quality of life for hospice patients and families.

The objective of this paper is to offer guidelines for tailoring key aspects of a foodservice operation to the inpatient hospice setting.

MENU PLANNING

As in any foodservice operation, in the hospice the menu is the hub of the system. It sets the stage for the equipment needed, space allocated, staff required, and budget expenditure. The menu is a communication medium to caregiving units outside the foodservice department (Sullivan, 1990). Therapeutically it offers the hospice patient an opportunity for choice when disease limits the opportunities for independence and control in many other aspects of life.

Primary to menu development is knowledge of the ethnic, cultural, and regional food preferences of the population. An understanding of an area's population mix, general food preferences of hospice patients, and routine menu and foodservice surveys provide the foodservice director with data. The regional daily meal pattern preference should also be considered. Should the menu reflect three meals, two lighter meals and one heavier meal, three meals with a heavy midday meal and a lighter evening meal, other combinations?

Regardless of meal pattern selected, there must be flexibility for re-heating menu items or preparing a quick meal when a hospice patient desires. Allowing patients to select menus as close to serving time as possible may help to allay the anorexia accompanying terminal illnesses. Small portions attractively garnished and plated in a dining atmosphere conducive to patient and family socialization also contribute to better patient meal acceptance. Family members' assistance with feeding further enhances the dining experience (Gallagher-Allred, 1989; National Cancer Institute, 1990).

In the hospice setting, many patients and families are concerned about whether the nutritional needs of the patient are being met. For example, some patients express a desire for additional fiber, others for low fat foods; still others for meals that reflect personal nutritional beliefs. Planning a menu based on the Basic Four Food Groups or the new USDA Food Guide Pyramid (Human Nutrition Information Service, 1992) will provide for nutritional adequacy. Specific dietary modifications, such as low sodium, low fat, and diabetic requirements also may be needed. In most hospice cases, however, these restrictions are liberalized to allow the patient maximum pleasure, variety, and choice.

Usually, menu planning focuses on the severity of patients' illnesses, the illness's impact on appetite and the need for food consistency modification. Fluctuations in patients' mental alertness, level of responsiveness, dental status, and swallowing difficulties may indicate the need for such consistency modifications as soft, mechanical soft, pureed, or blenderized foods.

Extensive menus with complicated, labor-intensive recipes should not be planned because these dishes are not well accepted nor well tolerated by patients with disease limitations. Simple, easy-to-prepare foods served in smaller portions are more acceptable to the hospice patient. "Comfort" or familiar foods are enjoyed and better tolerated. Some examples of universally selected comfort foods are macaroni and cheese, grilled cheese sandwiches, peanut butter and jelly sandwiches, meatloaf, soups, fresh fruits, and salads. These and other comfort foods of the geographic/cultural area or the particular patient should be considered when planning the hospice menu.

Patient length-of-stay will influence the number of weeks in the planned menu cycle. An acute care hospice with a seven day average length-of-stay will most likely use a one week cycle menu whereas a hospice with an average 28 day length-of-stay might use a four week cycle menu.

The following considerations for planning menus are vital for the success of the foodservice operation:

- What equipment is available for food preparation?
- What is the budget allowance for food, labor, and supplies?

- What are the availability and skills of foodservice production personnel?
- What type of production system (e.g., cook/serve, cook/chill, etc.) will be used?
- What type of tray delivery system will be used?
- What distance must the food be transported for service to the patient?
- How much space is available for food storage, preparation, and service?
- In what form will food be purchased–fresh, frozen, convenience, etc.?
- What type of menu will be used–selective, non-selective, cyclic, restaurant-style?
- Can the menu be adapted to seasonal and market conditions where popular menu items can be incorporated with cost-effectiveness?
- Does the menu balance production work-load from day-to-day?

Adequate menu preparation impacts on clinical patient care as well as on the foodservice aspects of hospice. A registered dietitian is trained to balance these factors in developing a menu that "works" for the individual hospice setting.

FOOD PURCHASING, STORAGE, AND PRODUCTION

Forecasting food supply needs in the hospice setting is difficult because of the seriousness of the patients' illnesses and rapid patient turnover. Some hospice dietitians have observed that patient census may remain stable but the ability of patients to eat fluctuates from a traditional meal pattern to only being able to tolerate small bites and sips. There are times when groups of patients have very good appetites and times when appetites generally are poor. When planning daily production quantities, the foodservice director/dietitian must regularly monitor census, patients' appetites and their ability to tolerate solid foods.

The next aspect of food production is purchasing food and supplies. The purchasing functions for a hospice unit that is located in a larger facility require no special considerations. The following discussion pertains to purchasing for a free-standing hospice.

In a Free-Standing Hospice

When purchasing food and supplies, for a free-standing hospice the foodservice director must first set standards for food quality and service. Based on these standards, she or he uses the menu and standardized recipes as a guide in determining quantities as well as quality. The availability of storage space, inventory levels, procedures for receiving, and vendors servicing the local area will also affect purchasing decisions. Since free-standing hospices produce a relatively smaller volume of meals daily and often have limited storage space, vendor selection may be limited. Selection of a local reliable vender who is capable of providing smaller package sizes and more frequent deliveries is essential. Also non-traditional supply sources such as local groceries may be needed for low use food products not available in split cases or individual units from vendors. In some communities purchases from a food-buying group or co-op may be an option.

Inventory

Purchasing schedules are specific to each hospice and will depend on the amount of storage space, menu, food production needs, vendors' service and delivery, availability of food, and cost. Some staples may need to be ordered on an infrequent basis while perishables may need to be ordered more often, perhaps two or three times per week.

The foodservice director must determine inventory levels and initiate and follow receiving and storage procedures. The cost of food, supplies, and small equipment—major segments of the hospice foodservice expenditure—may be controlled by avoiding either excessive or insufficient inventory levels, and by ensuring that goods on hand are stored in a secure place. There is continual need for the foodservice director to monitor and adjust food and supplies on hand to prevent irregularities. To operate efficiently and to compile accurate costs, the value and quantity of inventory items must be known. In a small hospice it is usually sufficient to make a visual check of items in the storeroom and main kitchen to determine purchasing needs.

A physical inventory is also necessary in calculating actual costs. For this purpose the storeroom should have a planned layout to facilitate regular visual surveys of stock levels and to plan reordering.

Fiscal Responsibility

Fiscal responsibility in the foodservice department requires a knowledge of all costs of foodservice operation. Data such as patient census, number of meals served, cost of food, supplies, small equipment, equipment maintenance, repair and replacement, and labor can be analyzed to determine daily food costs and other foodservice expenses. The foodservice director must develop monitoring tools to collect these data. Overall, the foodservice director in the free-standing hospice must exercise creativity in purchasing, storage, and production to achieve the standard of quality for meal service within budgetary guidelines.

TRAY DELIVERY AND DISTRIBUTION

Food delivery in a hospice usually follows a meal schedule typical of the particular region or culture, however, individual requests of terminally ill patients will require many modifications in this schedule. Some patients will sleep late and want a late breakfast, hence a late lunch and a late dinner as well. Others may want part of a meal at the usual time and the rest of it later. Illness, medications, and individual preferences play a major role in creating an unlimited schedule for meal times. The tray delivery system must accommodate these wishes at the same time it must ensure quality meals in microbiological safety. Pertinent questions to ask when considering what type of tray delivery system will be appropriate might be:

- Is food quality maintained?
- How long can food be maintained at safe temperatures by the system?

- Is the system compatible with the food production system?
- Can nursing staff and/or volunteers who often deliver meal trays use the system easily?
- Does the system physically fit into the existing kitchen and hospice environment?
- What is the cost of using and maintaining the system?
- Does the system require an energy source for maintaining temperatures? Is an outlet available in the kitchen and immediate hospice area?
- Are the cleaning and maintenance needs of the system compatible with the available staff and their skills?

Most tray delivery systems available today can be adapted for use in a hospice setting when the hospice is a physical part of a larger facility such as a long-term care or an acute care setting. However, it may be necessary for an independent hospice to narrow its choices to those systems that are the simplest and easiest to use and maintain. There are several basic types of systems that meet these criteria. Individual tray delivery systems that are well suited for the hospice setting are discussed below.

Insulated Tray System

The insulated tray system is a lightweight system with no special cart required for transport. However, the tray itself is bulky and may be cumbersome in its space requirements and storage. Special racks may be needed for the dishwasher.

Unitized Pellet System

The unitized pellet system uses a preheated pellet base and cover for the main plate to maintain hot food temperatures. For approximately 45 minutes insulated bowls and cups can be used for soups and hot liquids. Individual pellet lowerators, racks to hold covers, and insulated carts are required. The equipment is simple, easily portable, and requires only routine maintenance. It also affords flexibility in the hospice since meals that are going to be eaten later can be refrigerated and reheated in a microwave oven.

Other Systems

There are other systems that utilize hot and cold carts, but because electrical outlets are needed and more maintenance is required, they are more complex. These systems, useful when a hospice is a part of a larger organization, are not the most practical for a free-standing facility.

No matter what system is used, there must be procedures for ensuring that food temperatures are appropriately maintained. Nursing staff must be aware of how long trays can be held after delivery so they can refrigerate food that will not be used within this time period.

Tray Delivery on the Hospice Unit

Nursing staff and in some cases volunteers are responsible for delivering and handling meals once they arrive from the kitchen. This poses two major concerns for the foodservice manager. First, simple guidelines for food handling are needed to ensure food safety. This will be discussed in the section on inservice training. Second, a simple tray delivery system where food is heated and assembled prior to delivery will ensure accurate meal delivery with temperatures primarily controlled by the foodservice staff.

Managing Foods Brought into the Hospice from Home

Another aspect of hospice foodservice delivery is handling foods brought from home. While home food preparation cannot be monitored by the foodservice department, every effort should be made to provide on-site safe refrigerated storage and a re-heating system. This is accomplished by a family kitchen in the hospice unit. Rules for labeling and dating outside food items and safe storage time limits should be posted in the hospice kitchen. In addition, a policy may be established that outside food brought in for individual patients may not be shared with others because of contamination risks. Patient choice and willingness to accept this risk may be cause for exception.

PERSONNEL REQUIREMENTS

Another important aspect of a foodservice department in an inpatient hospice is that of staffing. This involves forecasting personnel needs, and the recruitment, selection, and training of employees. Additional staff may be needed if food will be offered to people other than patients (e.g., staff, family, volunteers, visitors) or if other foodservice functions such as catering are expected. Other considerations for staffing include the meal pattern, menu type, menu and recipe complexity, projected patient census, number and type of diet modifications, and amount of time available for menu preparation and service. Once these decisions are made, the foodservice director is ready to plan for the number of foodservice employees and the person-hour requirements necessary to accomplish the projected workload.

Staff Duties

Duties of staff will vary with the size of the hospice. There are many staffing combinations that can meet production needs. Cooks are central and their roles and responsibilities encompass more variation in duties and skills than in traditional settings. The cook's duties might encompass hot food production in addition to hot food plating; dining room hot foodservice as needed; and other cleaning and maintenance duties as directed in the job description and daily work schedule. The cook also has the responsibility of ensuring sanitation and safety of all aspects of food production. Other duties may include assisting with inventory and ordering. The cook's assistant or foodservice worker assists in other areas as needed by the foodservice department.

Small volume production may require only one cook and one cook's assistant and/or foodservice worker for each shift. Job interest and the desire to serve the needs of patients, families, friends, and the mission of the organization are necessary characteristics to consider when selecting the foodservice staff. It takes an exceptional employee to interrupt his/her routine to scramble an egg or make a sandwich at any time. This is one of many examples of the dedication of hospice foodservice workers.

FOOD SANITATION AND SAFETY

The hospice setting is one in which many patients are immune-compromised, hence vulnerable to infection. Therefore, a major responsibility of the foodservice department is to maintain the highest level of food sanitation and safety to prevent problems with food-borne pathogens and intoxicants. Understanding that microorganisms from man, animals, air, soil, water, and even the food supply itself are sources of contamination is essential to providing safe food.

The common food-borne illnesses result from the growth of bacterium, virus, or parasitic organisms in the gastrointestinal tract and usually manifest themselves within 8-72 hours depending on a variety of factors including the amount of toxin ingested and the susceptibility of the individual. *Salmonella, C. perfringens*, and *staphlococcus aureus* are the most common sources of food-borne illnesses. Specifics on the sources of contamination and symptoms of these diseases should be understood by all foodservice personnel. Primary prevention in each of these cases involves proper food handling, strict hand washing and personal hygiene, sanitary preparation of all foods throughout production processes, and maintenance of safe temperatures from the receipt of foods into the facility through their service (Longree & Armbruster, 1987).

The provision of safe food to a highly vulnerable hospice population not only involves a knowledge of the potential contaminants but also a thorough understanding of how microorganisms can be controlled in all phases of the foodservice operation including purchasing, receiving, storing, handling, processing, transporting, and serving. Standards for ensuring sanitary food handling have been developed by the Food and Drug Administration (FDA) in the Model Foodservice Sanitation Ordinance of 1976. This document was incorporated into the FDA Foodservice Sanitation Manual (Food and Drug Administration, 1978a) and has been adopted by many state and local health agencies.

Time and Temperature Relationships

Particularly for the hospice where flexibility in meal times may result in holding food for longer periods than usual, time and temperature relationships are paramount for food safety. Major emphasis should be placed on maintaining cold foods at less than 40°F (4.5°C) and hot foods at greater than 140°F (60°C) as illustrated in Figure 1. A guideline for timing in foodservice is that no more than two hours should elapse between preparation and service. This ensures food safety and protects the patient.

Care of Utensils

Lastly, the small free-standing hospice with limited space and resources has primary responsibility for cleaning and sanitizing dishes, utensils, and equipment. One should refer to his or her own state department of health rules and regulations for licensure, certification, and quality of care in establishing sanitation procedures. Suggested guidelines and warewashing equipment for this type of hospice follow.

Two types of dishwashers are recommended for the free standing hospice kitchen:

A. Single-tank, stationary rack, dual temperature machine with a wash temperature of 150°F (66°C) and a final rinse temperature of 180°F (82°C).

B. Single-tank, stationary rack, single temperature machine with both wash and final rinse temperatures of 165°F (74°C).

Basic guidelines for minimum temperatures for dishwashers are that the wash temperature should be at least 120°F (49°C) and the final rinse temperature with an approved chemical sanitizer, at least 75°F (24°C) (Puckett & Miller, 1988). Specific washing and sanitizing chemicals are approved by the state or local health authority. Following sanitizing, all washed items should be air-dried on drain boards or dish racks.

When there is no dishwasher or no washer for equipment and utensils, a 3-compartment sink is essential for washing, rinsing and sanitizing. Equipment and utensils should first be scraped and rinsed; then washed in a hot detergent solution in the first sink; rinsed with clean, hot water in the second sink; and finally sanitized using sanitizing chemicals and other methods approved by the local health authority. Cleaned dishes, equipment, and utensils should

FIGURE 1. Critical Temperatures in Sanitation and Food Safety

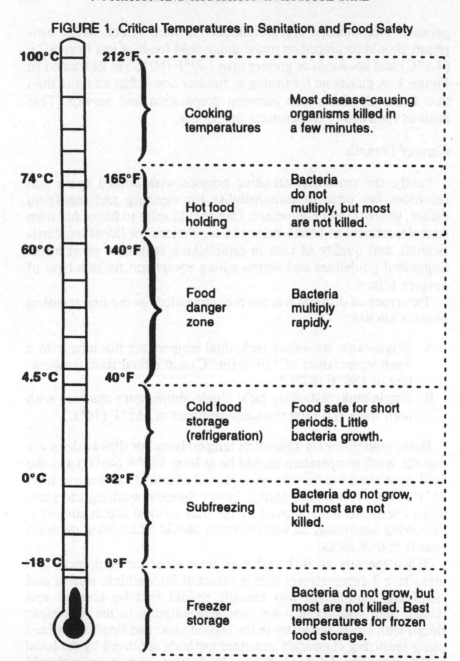

Note: Adapted form *Preventing Foodborne Illness: A Guide to Safe Food Handling* (USDA Home and Garden Bulletin No. 247 by Food Safety and Inspection Service, 1990, Washington, D.C.: U.S. Government Printing Office).

then be stored in a place at least six inches off the floor in a clean, dry, contaminant-free environment.

QUALITY CONTROL

The importance of sanitation and food safety is so significant in the hospice setting that quality control measures cannot be overlooked. One organized and comprehensive quality control method is the Hazard Analysis Critical Control Point modified by Bobeng and David (1978) for medical foodservice systems. This method directs monitoring of each of the critical steps in the foodservice operation where loss of control would jeopardize microbiological food safety. The four critical control points that must be monitored include: ingredient control and storage, equipment sanitation, personnel sanitation, and time-temperature relationships (Bobeng & David, 1978). The hospice foodservice manager must develop ways to check key aspects in each of these areas regularly. Simple ways to monitor these critical areas could be to check all temperatures in all food storage areas–refrigerated, frozen and dry storage–daily. A quick walk-through the kitchen with a focus on equipment sanitization between uses and hand-habits of foodservice staff could be used as key monitors for equipment and personnel sanitation. Lastly, temperature monitoring throughout food preparation, holding, assembly of trays, and service is critical. Food must not be held in a 40°F (4.5°C) to 140°F (60°C) zone where bacteria multiply quickly.

Food Quality and Acceptance

Another aspect of quality control is food quality and acceptance. After steps have been taken to ensure the highest standards of sanitation throughout food handling processes, quality control is mostly reliant on standardized recipes and recipe compliance. To monitor the quality of foods, the foodservice manager must develop product standards for them. These are written descriptions of appearance, texture, and flavor. Appendix C in the text by M. C. Spears (1991) provides a reference for common food product standards.

Patient Evaluation

Beyond intradepartmental quality evaluation is patient evaluation. This will provide the ultimate feedback on perceived food quality and acceptance. In the hospice setting, use of a simple meal evaluation survey with no more than three or four questions can provide the foodservice manager with invaluable feedback on food quality, the need for improvement, and most important whether meals are meeting patients' and families' expectations. Volunteers can assist the foodservice department in discussing these questionnaires with patients.

FACILITY LAYOUT AND EQUIPMENT SELECTION

Main Foodservice Area

The initial planning of the inpatient hospice unit may be as varied as the number of individual hospices themselves. There are in general two major types of inpatient setting—one part of a larger facility and the other free-standing. When a hospice is part of an acute or long-term care facility, the layout of the foodservice area is not a primary concern for the hospice unit. In the free-standing hospice, however, the foodservice director should be involved in the initial planning of the total facility. The foodservice director may be able to offer expertise in foodservice layout, space allocation, and departmental needs as they relate to the facility as a whole. In addition, the services of a foodservice design consultant may need to be used for more specific planning of an efficient, cost-effective operation (Birchfield, 1988).

Food Service Production System

Several other decisions should be made early in the planning phases of the foodservice operation. First, selection of a food production system for patients will dictate the kind and amount of equipment needed. There are four basic food production systems; cook and serve, cook and chill, cook and freeze, and assemble and serve. In meeting the needs of hospice patients, the cook and serve system is the most flexible. It offers greater menu variety and greater meal time adaptability. In addition, decisions need to be made whether others besides patients will be served, e.g., staff, volunteers, family, friends and/or others.

Equipment

Essential equipment depends on the menu pattern, selections offered, menu complexity, types of diets and modifications, types and numbers of meals prepared, and types of service. Table 1 outlines suggested equipment needs for a small independent hospice foodservice operation using the cook and serve system. When selecting foodservice equipment, every effort should be made to ensure that sanitary design, construction, and materials are durable, non-toxic, and capable of being cleaned and sanitized. Purchasing equipment that displays the seal of approval of the National Sanitation Foundation (NSF) or the Underwriters' Laboratory (UL) ensures the above criteria will be met.

Staff/Visitor Dining Room

Being able to offer the same menu items in another foodservice outlet such as a small dining room or a modified one room cafeteria is useful in meeting the needs of staff, volunteers, family, and visitors. A dining room/cafeteria is an effective way to utilize foods that have been prepared but not served for patient meals. This controls waste, decreases cost, and can be a source of revenue. This dining room/cafeteria located in a free-standing hospice can be operated by the same staff that prepares patient meals. In addition, this area offers a welcome place of respite for staff, family, friends, and volunteers.

This room is also adaptable. It can be incorporated in a free-standing hospice with a minimal amount of additional equipment. One of the many options would include using a small hot food cart and two or three long tables adapted to display other food items, service ware, coffee and beverage service, condiments, and paper products. Cold foods requiring refrigeration can be displayed in ice-filled containers. Several tables and chairs complete the furnishing of this dining environment.

TABLE 1. Suggested Equipment Needs for a Small Free-Standing Hospice Main Foodservice Area Using the Cook and Serve System

Major Equipment	Small Equipment
Range—may be a combination six or eight burner range with a broiler, grill and double ovens	Blender
	Food Processor
Refrigerator Unit(s)—reach-in or walk-in	Scales
	Toaster
Freezer Unit(s)—reach-in or walk-in	Coffeemakers
	Measurers
Microwave Oven	
Food Slicer	Pans
Dishwashing Machine	Knives
Disposal	Cutting Boards
Worktables	Thermometers
	Portioning Utensils
Mobile Equipment (Carts)	
	Cooking Utensils
Storage Shelves—for small equipment and utensils as well as for dry storage	Service Ware
	Flatware
Covered Waste Receptacles	Serving Utensils
Equipment for Tray Delivery System	Storage Containers
Cabinets/Dish Lowerator	

This room is also adaptable for other uses such as meetings, conference groups, and special functions during non-scheduled meal times. Simple decorating can be accomplished with the support of the community. For example, donations of garden flowers, plants, and perhaps even the loan of a local artist's works for exhibition can easily meet decorating needs.

Inpatient "Family" Kitchen Unit

Another essential component to the hospice environment and a satellite of the foodservice department is the inpatient kitchen unit or "family" kitchen. This unit is important as many patients have anorexia or decreased appetite and find small, frequent meals and small snacks throughout the day preferable to the traditional meal pattern. This kitchen may also stock foods as a medium for the administration of medications and should, in addition, contain liquids and ice for those patients unable to tolerate solid foods. The family kitchen offers families and friends a place to store and re-heat favorite foods brought in for the hospice patient. Hospice experience has shown that this type of kitchen is more efficient and cost-effective than a scheduled nourishment cart.

Organization of this family kitchen should be simple, incorporating principles of food sanitation and safety. Only the most basic equipment for storage and re-heating is necessary. Microwave ovens are safest and allow for the use of disposable plates, cups, and containers for cooking–all of which are more sanitary and easier to use in this environment. Kitchen ranges tend to be under-utilized and pots and pans may not be properly sanitized. In addition, ranges pose fire and safety hazards. Other equipment used in hospice family kitchens include a refrigerator with a large freezer, ice/water dispensing machine, toaster or toaster oven, blender, and coffee-maker.

The kitchen should also include a home-size sink with a garbage disposal. To comply with local health department regulations, a covered waste container is required and an additional handwashing sink with soap and disposable towel dispenser is usually needed. Sanitation standards can be ensured by using disposable service ware and plastic flatware.

To facilitate the smooth operation of this kitchen, the nursing and foodservice departments must post in a conspicuous place guidelines for its use, maintenance, and cleaning. Maintenance and cleaning responsibilities should be delegated as agreed upon by these two departments.

Food supplies for the family kitchen are determined by many factors including the type of patients, geographic and cultural influences, cost, ease of storage and sanitation requirements. Individually packaged, pre-portioned food items are convenient and ensure proper sanitation. Some of the frequently requested snack foods to include in a family kitchen are: fruit and vegetable juices, milk, ice cream, sherbet, fruit ices, puddings, crackers, peanut butter, jelly, bread, applesauce, cereals, and soups.

INSERVICE TRAINING NEEDS

All personnel–foodservice and non-foodservice including nursing and volunteer–using the kitchen must learn the basic aspects of sanitary and safe food handling as they apply to the hospice unit or family kitchen. A review of key concepts used for food handling in such a unit that might be covered in inservice training include:

- Food itself, food contact surfaces, food preparation equipment and the environment are sources of food contamination;
- Perishable food items must be held at temperatures outside the zone of 40°F (4.5°C) to 140°F (60°C) to minimize bacterial growth;
- The safe holding time of the current tray delivery system;
- Basic rules for food storage including proper temperatures for storing all types of foods, labeling and dating stored food items, and using separate storage areas for cooked and raw foods;
- Use of disposable heating containers, dishes, and tableware provides for maximum sanitation for patients and eliminates the need for washing and sanitizing between uses when time is limited.

Issues Surrounding AIDS

Another training issue for the foodservice staff is that of AIDS. Even though AIDS is not a food-borne illness, foodservice employees often express the fear that their contact with soiled dishes and tableware used by AIDS patients will put them at risk. "The Office of the U.S. Surgeon General and the Centers for Disease

Control (CDC) advise: (a) foodservice operations are safe places to work and dine, (b) AIDS cannot be passed through daily routines that occur in foodservice establishments, and (c) AIDS is not transmitted through food or drink" (National Restaurant Association, 1987). Therefore, the CDC does not recommend any special practices for food handling or for foodservice employees. Instead the CDC recommends that the usual food handling precautions be followed.

HOSPICE AS A PART OF A LONG-TERM CARE OR HOSPITAL SETTING

For most of its functions, a hospice within a larger institution is like other nursing units from the standpoint of foodservice. The institution's menu usually meets the needs of the hospice. However, flexibility of the foodservice department will be essential to provide special request items when possible. The institution's dietitian or dietetic technician will be helpful in utilizing his or her knowledge of the full menu and its modifications to provide patients with foods they are able to tolerate and enjoy. This may mean mixing food selections from various diets to meet the needs of a hospice patient.

Meal Ordering

Individual diets or meals are ordered by the hospice nursing staff using the same diet order requisition system as the rest of the institution. In the case of a long-term care facility where diets are not updated daily and only diet order changes are communicated to the foodservice department, the hospice will require at minimum a daily census and diet order requisition form to send to the foodservice department. Hospice nursing personnel can then make telephone updates to this list as necessary.

Meal Service

Depending on the institution, meal trays may be delivered to patients by foodservice staff or by nursing staff. When a patient does not want to eat at the usual meal time, the nursing staff takes the responsibility for holding the meal for the patient. Nourishments, snacks, and some comfort foods such as bouillon, instant hot cereal, juice, tea, ice cream, and fruit ices are conveniently stored in the hospice unit or family kitchen.

Stocking the Hospice Unit with Food Supplies

In most hospice units in larger institutions, the nursing staff is responsible for taking a daily inventory and ordering unit kitchen supplies using a nourishment/snack requisition form that is sent to the foodservice department. Ordering is easiest when supplies are replenished using an established "par level" for each food item. Special request items can also be written on this form. This is the easiest way to maintain an account for hospice unit supplies while allowing for changes in census and individual desires of patients residing in the hospice. As is the case with meal service, tube feedings and orders for special medical nutritional supplements are handled in the same manner as with any unit in that particular institution.

REIMBURSEMENT FOR NUTRITION
AND FOOD SERVICES IN HOSPICE

Reimbursement of nutrition and food services depends on the individual health insurance plans and whether a hospice is Medicare certified. In the Medicare certified hospice food services are covered as a core service under the bed and board provisions. Tube feedings and parenteral solutions are separately reimbursed as are drugs and other supplies. Nutrition counseling is explicitly cited along with physician, nursing, and social service as a core counseling service.

Medicaid is another source of reimbursement. The federal Medicaid guidelines do not specifically reference nutrition care, but give states authority to set eligibility criteria, coverage policies, and reimbursement methodologies. This means that Medicaid guidelines in each state must be analyzed to determine the extent of coverage and reimbursement for nutrition care services (American Dietetic Association, 1991).

In today's changing health care financing environment, practitioners need to pay special attention to legislation affecting the provision of food and nutrition services that can prevent undue suffering and improve a patient's quality of life.

CONCLUSION

By serving nutritious, attractively prepared food for visual and physical pleasure, the hospice foodservice staff has the opportunity to enrich patients' lives at a time when the smallest pleasure is truly treasured. This hospice philosophy as it affects foodservice is carried throughout all aspects of foodservice operations. Menu planning incorporates variety and comfort foods that satisfy patients' needs. Food production allows for flexibility in the scheduling and the serving of attractive meals. Foodservice facility layout, even though often compromised in terms of space, shows considerations for the adaptability needed in a hospice setting. A family kitchen further supports flexibility for meal service and supports family and friends in their caring efforts to nourish. Lastly, sanitation standards provide for the food safety required to ensure quality of life.

REFERENCES

Amenta, M. O., & Bohnet, N. L. (1986). *Nursing care of the terminally ill.* Boston: Little, Brown and Company.

American Dietetic Association (1991). *Reimbursement and insurance coverage for nutrition services.* 1989-90 Nutrition Services Payment Systems Committee. Chapter 2: Government Programs. Chicago: The American Dietetic Association.

Birchfield, J. C. (1988). *Design and layout of foodservice facilities.* New York: Van Nostrand Reinhold.

Bobeng, B. J., & David, B. D. (1978). HACCP models for quality control of entree production in hospital foodservice systems. I. Development of hazard analysis critical control point models. II. Quality assessment of beef loaves utilizing HACCP models. *Journal of the American Dietetic Association, 73* (5), 526.

Food and Drug Administration (1978). *A food service sanitation manual.* 1976 (revised). U.S. Dept. of Health Education and Welfare, Public Health Service, DHEW Publ. No. (FDA) 78-2081. Washington, D.C.

Gallagher-Allred, C., (1989). *Nutritional care of the terminally ill*. Rockville, MD: Aspen Publishers, Inc.

Human Nutrition Information Service (1992). *USDA's food guide pyramid*. (USDA Home and Garden Bulletin No. 249). Washington, DC: U.S. Government Printing Office.

Longree, K., & Armbruster, G. (1987). *Quantity food sanitation*. (4th ed.). New York: John Wiley & Sons.

National Cancer Institute. (1990). *Eating hints*. (NIH Publication No. 91-2079). Bethesda, MD: National Institutes of Health.

National Restaurant Association. (1987). *Basic facts about AIDS for foodservice employees*. Washington, DC: National Restaurant Association.

Puckett, R. P., & Miller, B. B. (1988). *Food service manual for health care institutions*. (1988 ed.). American Hospital Publishing, Inc.

Spears, M. C. (1991). *Foodservice organizations: A managerial and systems approach*. (2nd ed.). New York: Macmillan Publishing Co.

Sullivan, C. F. (1990). *Management of medical foodserservice*. (2nd ed.). New York: Van Nostrand Reinhold.

Enteral and Parenteral Nutrition Support of Terminally Ill Patients: Practical and Ethical Perspectives

Mark A. McCamish
Nancy J. Crocker

SUMMARY. The ethics of dealing with the provision of nutrition has been greatly complicated by technological advances. Seventy percent of all deaths in the United States include a decision to forgo some life-sustaining treatment including nutrition support. This article reviews ethical issues in nutrition support, appropriate and inappropriate nutrition support, practical information regarding provision of nutrition, and the development of institutional policies regarding artificial nutrition and hydration. Communication is emphasized in the process of establishing an ethically defensible consensus between patient and caregiver regarding withholding or withdrawing nutrition support. Within this context, withholding and withdrawing this support are considered to have the same ethical significance. Artificial nutrition and hydration is considered medical therapy and can be refused by competent patients and surrogates of

Mark A. McCamish, PhD, MD, is Director of Clinical and Metabolic Research at Ross Laboratories, and Clinical Associate Professor of Medicine at Ohio State University in Columbus, OH. Nancy J. Crocker, MS, RD, is a nutrition support team dietitian at the University of California, Davis, Sacramento Medical Center, Sacramento, CA.

Address correspondence to: Mark A. McCamish, PhD, MD, Ross Laboratories, Dept. 105600/RP3-2, 625 Cleveland Avenue, Columbus, OH 43215.

[Haworth co-indexing entry note]: "Enteral and Parenteral Nutrition Support of Terminally Ill Patients: Practical and Ethical Perspectives." McCamish, Mark A. and Nancy J. Crocker. Co-published simultaneously in *The Hospice Journal* (The Haworth Press, Inc.) Vol. 9, Nos. 2/3, 1993, pp. 107-129: and: *Nutrition and Hydration in Hospice Care: Needs, Strategies, Ethics* (eds: Gallagher-Allred, Charlette, and Madalon O'Rawe Amenta) The Haworth Press, Inc., 1993, pp. 107-129. Multiple copies of this article/chapter may be purchased from The Haworth Document Delivery Center [1-800-3-HAWORTH; 9:00 a.m. - 5:00 p.m. (EST)].

© 1993 by The Haworth Press, Inc. All rights reserved.

incompetent patients under certain circumstances. Patient autonomy is emphasized as a guiding ethical principle.

INTRODUCTION

The ethics of dealing with the provision of nutrition has been complicated by the increasing technological advances that have affected all of medical science. It is possible to totally support patients on artificial nutrition and hydration through either an enteral or parenteral route. The term artificial nutrition and hydration is used to connote provision of fluids and nutrient through any means other than spontaneous oral intake. This includes parenteral or IV infusions as well as other access routes such as nasogastric tubes.

Many patients can continue a successful work life even when they require parenteral nutrition through the use of home total parenteral nutrition (TPN) (Oley Foundation, 1985). Quality of life while providing prolonged life support, including the use of parenteral nutrition, follows a continuum from excellent to unacceptably miserable or useless (Angell, 1990; Luce, 1990; Smedira et al., 1990; Sprung, 1990; Uhlmann & Pearlman, 1991). This underscores the necessity of an ethical approach for decision-making regarding the initiation and continuation of artificial nutrition and hydration. Without a consistent approach, patients may end up as prisoners of technology (Angell, 1990).

PRACTICAL INFORMATION ON ARTIFICIAL NUTRITION AND HYDRATION

Once a patient is correctly identified as malnourished or at risk for malnutrition, a decision must be made regarding the use of nutrition support and the level of intervention. Can the patient be treated with diet alone, diet with supplements, tube feedings, or parenteral nutrition? Hospice programs provide enteral and parenteral nutrition support to dying patients. Examples of hospice patients for whom enteral or parenteral feedings are appropriate may include:

- those who have a feeding tube or line in place and want it used (e.g., patients with ALS or head and neck cancer);
- those for whom an untimely and uncomfortable death may occur without enteral or parenteral nutrition;
- those for whom it is important to prolong life so that an important event can occur before the patient dies (e.g., to attend a grandchild's graduation or wedding or to get business affairs in order);
- those for whom there is a threat of legal action if the tube/line is not placed or used when the patient's wishes are not known;
- those for whom the tube/line is a source of control or denial.

Once a decision is made to use nutrition support, one must identify the extent of gut function. This usually can be determined clinically. The rule of thumb is: if the gut functions, use it! Overall, if a patient has a soft abdomen with normal bowel sounds and has bowel movements or flatulence, this indicates bowel function. Nausea, vomiting, steatorrhea, diarrhea, or malabsorption may indicate some degree of dysfunction. Alternatively, a patient may have adequate gut function but be unable to chew or swallow.

Four Levels of Nutrition Intervention

Dietary Intervention

Many patients who are identified as malnourished have adequate gut function. Successful interventions to achieve adequate intake may include simply providing full meals and extra snacks, modifying the texture of food, or increasing nutrient density. Diets can be modified in terms of calorie, fat, and protein content to meet clinical needs. Intake and serial weights can be documented to ensure the patient is meeting appropriate nutritional goals. For more information, please refer to "Nutrition and Hydration in the Terminally Ill Cancer Patient" in this volume. That article contains suggestions for improving oral intake and treating anorexia and cachexia in terminally ill patients.

Patients and families should also be reassured that they are not guilty of having caused the illness through what the patient did or did not eat. An important goal for hospice patients is to enjoy any foods that are desired. In order to promote dignity in death, it is important to alleviate the patient's or caregiver's fear that they are responsible for the patient's demise.

Enteral Supplements

Enteral products, either commercial or homemade, can be used to augment the diets of patients who are malnourished but have adequate gut and deglutition function. Optimally, the diet would be supplemented by, not replaced with, the enteral product. Many patients who tire easily and do not have the strength to do much food preparation can use commercial supplements to conserve energy for other activities without sacrificing adequate nutritional intake.

Tube Feeding

When gut function is present but the patient cannot spontaneously take in adequate oral nutrition, tube feedings can be useful in prolonging meaningful life. Tube feedings are also essential to the support of life in patients in a persistent vegetative state (PVS) who can neither feed themselves nor take food orally, and who may be receiving palliative care. Enteral feedings can be provided as boluses throughout the day, as continuous infusions over 24 hours, or as nocturnal infusions to supplement the patient's spontaneous but inadequate daytime oral intake. As with any form of medical therapy, enteral tube feedings require informed consent. Also, for self-administration the patient or caregiver must be adequately trained to administer the feedings and troubleshoot complications. A registered dietitian and nurse should design the feeding protocol, provide training, and help monitor for complications.

Many enteral formulas have been compounded to provide a wide variety of features. There are formulas that vary in energy density from 1 kcal per cc (1 kilocalorie equals 1 food Calorie) to 2 kcals per cc. Others vary in protein content from approximately 15% to 22% of kcals. Some contain fiber and others are fiber-free.

Enteral products can generally be categorized into the following areas: (a) intact, (b) defined peptide, (c) elemental, and (d) disease-specific.

Intact products. These products contain whole proteins, complex starch, and long-chain triglycerides. They require complete endogenous digestion for absorption. These formulations can be used in most clinical situations unless there is significant stress, trauma, or limited gut function. They are the standard products used for hospice patients. Examples include Ensure, Ensure Plus, Sustacal, and Sustacal HC. These products, which are sweetened and come in a variety of flavors for oral use, can also be used for tube feedings. Nonflavored products such as Osmolite or Isocal, normally used for tube feedings, can be flavored with small amounts of syrups or other flavorings for oral use if other mixtures prove to be too sweet. Fiber-containing products may be useful when increasing stool bulk is desirable; e.g., in patients who are immobilized.

Intact products are less expensive than defined peptide, elemental, and disease-specific ones. Therefore, the need to use any of the specialized formulations should be evaluated for cost-effectiveness.

Defined peptide. These products contain hydrolyzed components that require less endogenous digestion. Hydrolyzed protein, which has shorter peptide chains, tri- and dipeptides as well as fat in long chain triglycerides are utilized. These products may be helpful during severe stress or when the patient's digestive and absorptive functions are insufficient to handle the intact products. Hospice patients who may benefit from defined peptide formulas include those with conditions such as malabsorption due to pancreatic cancer, liver cancer, radiation enteritis, and AIDS.

Elemental products. These preparations contain free amino acids as the protein source and a minimal amount of lipid to provide essential fatty acids. Their osmolarity is usually increased because of the monomeric amino acids and high carbohydrate content. Although the indications for elemental diets are the same as for defined peptide diets, there is limited scientific support for use of a truly elemental diet in hospice care as well as in critical care. Defined peptide products lead to more efficient absorption/utilization of protein or nitrogen (Keohane, Brown, & Grimble, 1981; Silk, Fairclough, & Clark, 1980). Note: many manufacturers now refer to their defined peptide products as "elemental" even though they do not have predominantly monomeric amino acids or minimal fat.

Disease-specific. Disease-specific products are tailored to provide more optimal nutrition support during specific disease states. There are disease-specific products that can be taken orally or used in tube feedings for the support of patients with diabetes, pulmonary disease, renal disease, and gastrointestinal insufficiency.

Because of the variety of available enteral products, a simple evaluation of the nutritional needs of the patient should be done to select the one most suited to the patient's needs and ability to pay. Since colonic microflora are generally affected by major changes in nutrient ingestion, it should be noted that one may experience constipation and/or diarrhea when adapting to sole source enteral nutrition or changing formulas.

Parenteral Nutrition

Parenteral nutrition is usually reserved for those at risk for malnutrition who have limited or no gut function or for those who have malnutrition that contributes to poor quality of life. Monomeric nutrients, such as glucose, amino acids, and micronutrients are infused directly into a vein, thus bypassing the gastrointestinal tract. Parenteral infusions, usually in the form of nutritionally-complete TPN, are used in hospice care to provide comfort and strength. If simple hydration is the major concern, however, peripherally-infused solutions providing only fluid and electrolytes should be used.

SPECIFICS OF NUTRITION SUPPORT

Enteral Nutrient Requirements

Water

Probably the most important and often overlooked nutrient, especially in geriatric patients, is water. Amongst the elderly, dehydration, the identification of which is difficult, is the most common fluid and electrolyte disorder (Lavizzo-Mourey, Johnson, & Stolley, 1988). Unrecognized and untreated dehydration can also complicate chronic medical problems and increase morbidity. Four factors are associated with inadequate fluid intake: speech difficulties, visual impairment, infrequent opportunities for water ingestion, and reduced time of availability of water during any 24-hour period (Mahowald & Himmelstein, 1981).

For practical purposes, water intake should parallel energy expenditure. Recommended requirements for adults are 1.0 to 1.5 mL of water per kcal of energy expended (Gaspar, 1988). Since energy needs in the elderly decrease over time, if the patient does not have a history of fluid overload or congestive heart failure, the requirement of 1.0-1.5 mL per kcal should cover variations in activity level, sweating, and solute load. It is important to realize, however, that the amount of free water in enteral products is not equivalent to the amount of total product infused. Free water, generally listed on the can, will vary depending on nutrient density. An eight oz. can (approximately 235mL) of a common enteral product (Ensure, Ross Laboratories, Columbus, OH) contains 200 mL of free water.

Sometimes it may be appropriate to provide enteral or parenteral feedings that only approximate an imminently dying patient's insensible fluid loses (500-600cc/day). This will be sufficient to prevent the over hydration that can cause loud "death rattle." It will also contribute to family comfort that hydration was maintained and dehydration was not painful.

Kilocalories/Energy

Providing 30-35 kcals of nutrition per kilogram body weight will be more than adequate in the general population. In the elderly nonambulatory population, caloric equilibration can occur at much lower levels such as 20-25 kcals per kilogram. For the hospice patient whose goal it is to maintain/improve strength, 25-30 kcals/ kg body weight is appropriate.

When providing artificial nutrition and hydration, a nutritional prescription should be implemented and the patient followed to determine whether goals are being met. However, weight and lab data are not generally monitored unless the benefits of having the data outweigh the burdens of collecting it, that is if the result will improve treatment, or the patient/family wants the information. The goal for hospice patients generally is to consume enough kcals to maintain or improve strength; not to achieve an ideal body weight. When the goal of maintaining or improving strength is not being met, the nutritional treatment–enteral or parenteral–can ethically be discontinued with the consent of the patient and/or family. Specific guidelines for implementation and monitoring can be found elsewhere (Rombeau & Caldwell, 1984, 1990).

Protein

The Food Nutrition Board Recommended Dietary Allowance for protein in healthy adults and the elderly population is 0.75 g of protein per kilogram of body weight (National Research Council, 1989). In reality, when providing a nutrition prescription, it is anticipated that individuals will not receive 100% of their prescription at all times, therefore, prescriptions are often increased by about 10%. Optimally, provision will approximate 0.8 to 1 g of protein per kilogram per day. Although achieving this protein intake with enteral or parenteral nutrition is relatively easy, with oral intake it may be difficult.

The overall goal in hospice care is physical and psychological strength. For patients with a limited life expectancy, physical strength is associated more with kilocalorie intake than with protein intake. Therefore, there is rarely a pressing need to provide high levels of protein in these situations and high protein intake will rarely improve a serum albumin level in a hospice patient.

Terminally ill patients who are able to take foods by mouth often dislike the taste of high-protein foods and may tolerate them better if they are served cold rather than hot, probably because they have less odor when cold. Best-liked protein-containing foods include eggs, chicken, fish, and dairy products.

Carbohydrate

Carbohydrates, basic source of fuel for some tissues and cells, can spare muscle and visceral protein from being oxidized for fuel. There is no recommended goal for carbohydrate intake except the provision of a sufficient amount to prevent ketosis (> 100 g/day) and to supply energy needs without stimulating hyperglycemia. In patients with known diabetes or hyperglycemia, simple carbohydrate intake can be decreased through many avenues including the use of enteral products specifically designed for diabetics. Carbohydrates are generally well-tolerated by terminally ill patients, and should be encouraged especially when protein tastes abnormal or when fat is not tolerated (e.g., because liver or pancreatic function is compromised).

Fat/Lipid

Essential fatty acid requirements can be met by providing 2%-3% of total kcals in the form of these lipids. It is relatively easy to meet the essential fatty acid requirements when utilizing any form of artificial nutrition and hydration including parenteral nutrition. Various enteral products may contain anywhere from 3% up to 55% of total kcal from fat. There is, therefore, a large variability in the specific amounts of carbohydrate and fat that may be provided to each patient. The recommendations of the American Heart Association, with its goal of preventing coronary heart disease, do not apply to hospice patients. Hospice staff should ask patients if they are avoiding foods high in fat and cholesterol in order to follow a "prudent" diet, since doing so in terminal illness is not only unnecessary but may be deleterious.

Vitamins/Minerals

The general requirements for vitamins and minerals, well-outlined in the National Research Council Recommended Dietary Allowances (National Research Council, 1989), need not be repeated here. What needs to be emphasized is the concern about vitamin/ mineral adequacy in terminally ill patients who have a relatively long life expectancy, or who are receiving enteral/parenteral nutrition support. Patients who have tried macrobiotic or other severely restrictive diets might well become deficient in many vitamins and/or minerals. Even in these cases high doses of supplemental vitamins/minerals are rarely necessary. One exception may be the use of Vitamin C and zinc supplements (less than $5 \times$ the Recommended Daily Allowances [USRDA's]) for malnourished terminally ill patients with pressure ulcers who are unable to maintain adequate oral intake. Vitamin or mineral toxicities may be a problem in hospice patients who have tried unorthodox nutrition therapies (e.g., megadoses of vitamin A, C, and beta carotene for various diseases).

When enteral formulas are used as a sole source of nutrition most are compounded to meet vitamin and mineral needs. The volume that provides 100% of the USRDA's is called the nutrient base volume and is generally listed. This information becomes useful when attempting to provide a full complement of nutrients without inducing continual weight gain if caloric needs should be limited due to inactivity. Nutrient-dense products (base < 1500mL) can be used or, if the patient can take medications by mouth, a vitamin/mineral supplement can be used. If energy expenditure is limited, a product with a relatively higher protein to kcal ratio may be helpful. In this way, the continued protein, vitamin, and mineral requirements can be met with a smaller caloric provision. (An example of such a product is Promote, Ross Laboratories, Columbus, OH.)

Fiber

Fiber may be important in two ways: (1) as a mechanism for water absorption and increasing stool bulk, and (2) as a fermentation agent in the colon providing specific nutrients (short-chain fatty acids) to help maintain optimal mucosal integrity of the colon. Fiber-containing formulas may be especially helpful for comatose or inactive patients in whom adequate fluid and fiber are needed to prevent or treat constipation or diarrhea.

A high percentage of hospice patients have pain that is controlled with narcotics, which also can cause constipation. A high fiber/high fluid diet, although sometimes difficult to spontaneously consume, is helpful in this situation as are stool softeners for preventing or treating constipation. If long-term enteral feeding is utilized as the sole source of nutrition then a fiber-containing product is a reasonable choice.

Parenteral Nutrient Requirements

Parenteral nutrition is markedly more complex and should be administered under the direction of clinicians and home healthcare personnel familiar with its use. In general, nutrient requirements can be met with parenteral nutrition compounded in one container that can be infused over a 12- to 24-hour period. These solutions contain crystalline amino acids as "protein," dextrose monohydrate as carbohydrate, and lipids in an emulsion of triglycerides, glycerol, and phospholipid. Trace minerals and vitamins are provided as combination mixtures that can be added by the pharmacy during compounding, or later if a week's supply of parenteral nutrition is delivered all at one time to the patient.

The following criteria should be met for instituting parenteral feedings in home care hospice patients: (1) patient consent, (2) adequate insurance coverage for supplies and skilled professional care, (3) presence of an appropriate and skilled care giver, and (4) venous access for a permanent central line catheter (Lin, 1991).

Monitoring

Each hospice program, institution, and home healthcare agency, as well as nutrition team, must establish its own comprehensive monitoring program. Guidelines for preventing complications and monitoring progress toward meeting nutritional goals should be developed. For example, the many serious complications associated with enteral feedings result from a displaced feeding tube. Guidelines should be in place to ensure that the enteral access device (e.g., nasoenteral tube) has not been displaced prior to the infusion of nutritional products.

Nasoenteral and nasogastric feeding tubes can be pulled out of position inadvertently by either patient or staff, or can migrate upward with vigorous coughing or vomiting. Unfortunately, these feeding tubes can also be displaced into the posterior oral pharynx, providing a route for aspiration of enteral formula into the lungs.

Auscultation is not a recommended method for assessing tube placement; aspiration of gastric contents is more accurate. Confirmation of nasal and percutaneous placements of duodenal or jejunal tubes generally requires radiologic documentation. Nasally placed tubes should be marked with permanent marker, if not done so by the manufacturer, proximal to the nares. Position of the mark should be noted and monitored to document tube migration. Provided this mark appears in the same location, displacement of the feeding tube since its last use is unlikely unless the patient has been vomiting or coughing vigorously. Other indicators to monitor include GI tolerance and hydration as well as weights and laboratory values such as serum electrolytes, if appropriate.

Monitoring should be intensive and frequent with parenteral nutrition because of its inherent associated risks of line sepsis and metabolic abnormalities. Central access site, temperature, weights, and metabolic/nutritional laboratory values must be carefully followed.

ARTIFICIAL NUTRITION AND HYDRATION: OPTIONS FOR ADMINISTRATION

Enteral

Nutrition support can be provided with supplements between meals, enteral products taken spontaneously by mouth, tube feedings provided as bolus or continuous feedings, and parenteral nutrition provided continuously or cycled on and off in various schedules. Bolus feedings should be used only when gastric access is available. They should not be administered directly into the small intestine. The gastric bolus size can be increased per patient tolerance until adequate nutrition is provided in five to six boluses throughout the day.

Some hospice patients may wish to take their tube feeding as bolus feeds at regular mealtimes. Similarly, care givers may wish to give bolus feeds to comatose or semi-comatose patients when the care givers eat their family meal. Bolus feeds may be viewed as symbolic of a normal meal, especially when the patient is in the same room with the family at the mealtime. Either continuous or nocturnal enteral tube feedings can provide artificial nutrition and hydration depending upon the desire and ambulatory capabilities of the patient.

Parenteral

Parenteral nutrition can be infused over 24 hours with momentary interruptions only to change infusion bags. Cyclical parenteral nutrition, however, is the usual mode of parenteral nutrition support for homecare and ambulatory patients. In this method, parenteral nutrition is cycled off and on to allow the patient freedom from the infusion apparatus for part of the day. Patients are hooked up to their IV access catheter and parenteral nutrition is infused, titrating up on the rate of infusion to prevent hyperglycemia. Once a constant rate of infusion is reached, it is maintained for approximately 8 to 10 hours when the infusion is then titrated back down over the last 1- to 2-hour period to prevent reactive hypoglycemia. Parenteral nutrition is then discontinued and the central line is flushed and capped until use the following day.

Education

It is imperative that a nurse and dietitian provide training to the family in the administration of artificial nutrition and hydration with emphasis on the prevention of complications. For example, enteral feeding tube clogging is a major problem that may require replacement of the nasoenteral access device. Tube clogging can be minimized by using frequent water flushing during and after feedings, and especially before and after administration of medications. Inappropriate manipulation of intravenous catheters used for TPN can result in infections, clotting, or air embolism.

APPROPRIATE AND INAPPROPRIATE USES OF ENTERAL AND PARENTERAL NUTRITION IN THE TERMINALLY ILL

The guidelines of The American Society of Parenteral and Enteral Nutrition (ASPEN) cite indications for the use of parenteral nutrition. The clinical situations in which parenteral nutrition should not be used include: (1) patients with functional and useable GI tracts, and (2) when sole dependency on parenteral nutrition is anticipated to be less than five days. The ASPEN guidelines also outline clinical situations in which parenteral nutrition is of limited value: (1) minimal stress and trauma in the well-nourished patient, (2) immediate post-operative and post-stress periods, and (3) proven or suspected untreatable disease states. These proscriptions are due intrinsically to the expense of parenteral nutrition and to the complications that can occur in providing venous access as well as to the metabolic and infectious complications that can arise from its administration.

There are also complications associated with the use of enteral nutrition. Many arise from failed or misguided attempts to provide enteral access. Complications can occur in the placement of naso-gastric and nasoenteral tubes as well as in the placement of longer term enteral access devices such as percutaneous endoscopic gastrostomies (PEG) or percutaneous endoscopic jejunostomies (PEJ). Nasoenteral feeding tubes can be misguided during initial placement into the pulmonary architecture permitting either infusion of enteral product into the lungs or directly causing mechanical damage such as pneumo- or hemothorax. Although these complications are infrequent, one should discuss them as possibilities when obtaining informed consent. It is, therefore, a mistake to consider either enteral or parenteral nutrition to be risk-free. These technologies should not be employed in the absence of a justified clinical rationale.

The Issue of Futility

When addressing inappropriate use of any medical technology including artificial nutrition and hydration, one should consider whether the therapy is futile. If provision of nutritional support imposes a severe burden on the patient, or if the patient will not actually benefit from such treatment, the effort can be determined futile. The concept of futility should be applied cautiously, however, since a possibly helpful medical therapy may not be offered and might even be withheld if it is deemed not beneficial (Singer & Siegler, 1991; Stanley, 1989).

The way in which a clinician defines futility, therefore, is important. It is important to establish not only the probability that the nutritional intervention will be successful, but also the goals by which success will be measured (Singer & Siegler, 1991). Since decisions regarding provision, withholding, or withdrawal of artificial nutrition and hydration may be unsettling or very painful, a time-limited trial may help in this sort of evaluation (The Hastings

Center, 1987). When a clear benefit versus burden decision cannot be determined, the less serious error calls for continued nutritional support until a decision can be made. The medical legal literature provides numerous examples of cases where patients may not be best served by nutritional support (Luce, 1990; Oley Foundation, 1985; Smedira et al., 1990).

WITHDRAWING OR WITHHOLDING ARTIFICIAL NUTRITION AND HYDRATION

The decision to withdraw or withhold nutrition or hydration life support is generally a difficult one unless the patient meets brain death criteria (President's Commission, 1981). In this case the patient is legally dead and all life support including artificial nutrition and hydration can be withdrawn. In all other situations, the principles of medical ethics can assist in these difficult decisions. Guiding ethical principles of withdrawing or withholding nutrition support have been extensively outlined elsewhere (Young, Perkins, & McCamish, 1992).

When dealing with the ethics of withdrawal of nutrition support, three questions should be addressed (Young et al., 1992): (1) Is artificial nutrition/hydration considered medical therapy? (2) Can competent patients refuse artificial nutrition/hydration? (3) Can an incompetent patient have artificial nutrition/hydration withdrawn based on a surrogate's request? Although case law at this time does not supply definitive answers to these three questions, the recent Nancy Cruzan case provides insights (Supreme Court Opinions, 1991).

In the Cruzan decision, the United States Supreme Court adopted the "consensus opinion that treats artificial nutrition and hydration as a medical treatment" (*Nancy Beth Cruzan v. Director*, 1990, p. 7136). Most experts in this area also believe that provision of artificial nutrition and hydration is not distinguishable in a morally relevant way from other life-sustaining treatments (Singer & Siegler, 1991; Sprung, 1992).

For the purposes of the Cruzan case, the court also "assumed that a competent person would have a constitutionally protected right to refuse life-sustaining hydration and nutrition" (*Nancy Beth Cruzan v. Director*, 1990, p. 7136).

Regarding the third question–withdrawal of artificial nutrition/ hydration at surrogate's request–Missouri had recognized that under certain circumstances a surrogate may decide to have artificial nutrition and hydration withdrawn in such a way as to allow death, but the state established a procedural safeguard. The procedural safeguard involved principles of evidentiary law in that Missouri required "clear and convincing" evidence that Nancy Cruzan would refuse artificial nutrition and hydration. This is the highest level of evidence and generally requires direct testimony of specific conversations with the patient or written prior directives. The U.S. Supreme Court ruled that this safeguard was not unconstitutional.

In other words, Missouri could refuse to grant withdrawal of nutrition and hydration if the patient's desire was not demonstrated with "clear and convincing" evidence. The U.S. Supreme Court did not rule that it was unconstitutional to withdraw nutrition and hydration from Nancy Cruzan and eventually it was withdrawn leading to her death. The answer, therefore, to all three of the above questions is yes, under certain circumstances.

It is necessary to emphasize that, in circumstances where the patient expires when artificial nutrition and hydration is withdrawn, the cause of death is the underlying disease or condition, not the withdrawal of the nutrition support. Many clinicians and ethicists, clearly distinguishing between "killing" versus "allowing to die" (Institute of Medical Ethics, 1991; Luce, 1990; Raffin, 1991; Singer & Siegler, 1991), maintain that withdrawing nutrition and hydration falls into the "allowing to die" category. In the past, prior to the availability of advanced nutrition and hydration support technology, similar patients would have died of their disease. Advances in artificial nutrition and hydration technology have not changed this and, therefore, absence of nutrition support is not the specific cause of death.

This concept is very important to emphasize with patients, patient surrogates, and especially patients' families. Families already carry a sufficiently heavy burden without adding to it the burden of guilt due to a decision to withdraw artificial nutrition and hydration. Within the same context, "withholding" and "withdrawing" artificial nutrition and hydration are considered to have the same ethical significance (Luce, 1990; President's Commission, 1983; Raffin, 1991), even though the removal of artificial nutrition and hydration may be psychologically and emotionally much more difficult. This should not, however, lead to withholding this therapy in an attempt to avoid a difficult decision regarding withdrawing support in the future. Figure 1, an adaptation from Young, Perkins, and McCamish (1992), can serve as a general guideline in these matters.

GUIDELINES FOR DECISIONS TO WITHDRAW/ WITHHOLD ARTIFICIAL NUTRITION SUPPORT

First, it is very important to establish the clinical facts regarding each patient's situation so that these can be effectively communicated to the patient, surrogate, and/or family. This information should include discussion of the benefit and/or burden the patient may experience with the therapy. Essential questions to be considered in provision of artificial nutrition and hydration relate to the concept of proportionality; that is, from the patient's perspective, will the potential benefits be greater than the burdens? The patient's educated perspective should be the cornerstone of the decision-making process. Always keep in mind that both parenteral and enteral nutrition are associated with complications, some of which can be severe. Note also that terminally ill patients who are dehydrated or malnourished are not necessarily uncomfortable. Forced hydration or nutrition may actually exacerbate problems in some cases. Therefore, if the patient will not clearly benefit from this treatment, the efforts may be considered futile.

Patient Autonomy and Informed Consent in Decision Making

The American Dietetic Association states that forgoing or discontinuing aggressive nutrition support may be considered when a competent patient wants it stopped, simply on the grounds that the patient perceives it as undignified, degrading, and physically or emotionally unacceptable (American Dietetic Association, 1992). Indeed, one of the most important guiding ethical principles is

FIGURE 1. Guidelines for Decisions to Withdraw/Withhold Artificial Nutrition Support

Autonomy

Does Patient Have Decisional Capacity? — No → Durable Power of Attorney or Prior Directive? — No → Identify Surrogate

Yes / Yes → Establish Ethically Defensible Consensus

Establish Clinical Facts/Disclosure
- Reasonable hope of benefit?
- Persistent vegetative state?
- Reasonable hope of regaining consciousness?

Maintain Integrity of Healthcare Professional
- Optimize interpersonal communication
- Personal moral or religious convictions violated?

Establish Ethically Defensible Consensus

Establish Pertinent Ethical/Legal Issues
- Undue, disproportionately great burden to:
  - Patient?
  - Family?
- Disproportionate social consequences? (Social Justice)
- Beneficence
- Nonmaleficence

Withhold/Withdraw Nutrition Support?

patient autonomy, or the right of each person to make decisions regarding her or his medical care, including refusal of treatment. Respect for this principle will lead to less intense clashes over patient wishes versus physician views regarding the patient's best interest (Lowe, Rouse, & Dornband, 1990).

Patients and family members want to be involved in medical decision making (Lowe, McLeod, & Saika, 1986). The patient, the family, the patient's physician, and other professionals involved in his or her care should communicate and collaborate in decision-making. Informed consent entails the physician's obligation to provide the competent patient with the information needed to make decisions regarding medical care. It is then the right of the competent adult patient to accept or refuse this treatment (Luce, 1990; Ruark & Raffin, 1988).

This process includes evaluating the patient's decision making capacity and, if necessary, a search for prior directives. If the patient does not have adequate decision-making capacity and a prior directive is not in effect, a surrogate must be identified. Unresolved questions and issues may indicate the need for outside evaluation either by an institution's ethics committee or legal affairs office.

Importance of Thorough Communication

Communication is the operational word. These difficult decisions are facilitated by effective communication with the patient or the patient's surrogate, family members, and other involved care givers. The goal is to identify the patient's wishes in each clinical situation, not what the healthcare professionals' wishes would be if they were in the same situation. If the patient's or surrogate's ethically justified decision is to refuse or to withdraw from the therapy, then the healthcare professional should comply. If healthcare professionals cannot comply due to personal, moral, or religious convictions, it is reasonable to transfer the patient's care to another professional practitioner who can (Young et al., 1992).

An additional consideration is that traditional clinicians with their science-based training believe that an answer can be determined if adequate facts are obtained. This may generate a seemingly never-ending process of garnering more facts and asking more questions. Ethical decisions, however, are often impossible to arrive at solely on the basis of facts. It cannot be overemphasized that establishing clinical facts is necessary but not sufficient–the principles of patient autonomy and clear communication are also critical elements in the process of discovering an ethically defensible consensus.

Legal Considerations

Although legal matters will be discussed elsewhere in this volume it is important to note here that if a medical care provider wishes to guarantee immunity from criminal prosecution, professional discipline, or liability damages regarding termination of life-sustaining therapy, she or he must follow the applicable state's statutes regarding advance directives. States differ, and the statutes and regulations of some are more complex than those of others. Since the legal system often trails technologic innovation, following the letter of the law will not prevent ethical dilemmas. From an ethical standpoint, the Hastings Center has advocated avoidance of routine judicial involvement if at all possible in these complex decisions (The Hastings Center Guidelines for Foregoing Treatment, 1988). Finding an ethically defensible consensus should be the goal.

In further emphasizing avoidance of routine judicial involvement, The Hastings Center Guidelines for Foregoing Treatment (1988) address surrogate identification when a patient is incapacitated. The clinician should first choose the individual designated by the patient in written or oral advance directives. If there is no advance directive and no court-appointed surrogate, the clinician should choose a close family member or friend. The goal is to identify the individual who is "most knowledgeable about the patient's present and past feelings and preferences" (p. 6).

Finally, an ethically defensible consensus regarding withholding or withdrawing artificial nutrition and hydration should be established. The end result is not to determine what is right or wrong in each particular case, but to establish an ethically defensible consensus. The clinical facts can be identical in two separate cases, yet due to issues of patient autonomy and evaluation of burden versus benefit, the ultimate decision may be exactly the opposite. As long as there is an ethically defensible consensus as previously outlined, neither decision can be called wrong.

DEVELOPING INSTITUTIONAL POLICIES ON ARTIFICIAL NUTRITION AND HYDRATION

In considering an institutional policy on artificial nutrition and hydration, a review of the Hospice of Washington's policy (Koshuta, Schmitz, & Lynn, 1991) is recommended. Since 70% of all deaths in the United States include a deliberate decision to forgo some life-sustaining treatment (President's Commission, 1981), it is reasonable to consider establishment of a policy regarding use of artificial nutrition and hydration. It is not necessary for this policy to be specific in treatment plans or to list which therapies can or cannot be withdrawn. A paragraph from the Hospice of Washington's discussion illustrates this point:

> Other than the refusal to deliberately end a patient's life, and our commitment to enhance life whenever possible, we have no policy which requires or bars any particular interventions. The care plan for each patient is developed and adjusted in collaboration with the patient, the patient's family and friends and the hospice staff, and is expected to reflect the individual patient's goals, values, and capabilities, and the professional expertise and personal commitment of the Hospice staff. (p. 138)

This policy was established by the Hospice of Washington for many reasons, but two important factors involved: (1) those patients and/or families who feared that the Hospice of Washington never allowed artificial nutrition and hydration, and (2) those who were seeking out Hospice of Washington on the assumption that they would automatically discontinue these treatments (Koshuta et al., 1991).

We have the technology to provide the very best nutrition support in most clinically appropriate situations. The information herein should stimulate evaluation of this technology so that we are justified in its use.

REFERENCES

American Dietetic Association. (1992). Position of the American Dietetic Association: Issues in feeding the terminally ill adult. *Journal of the American Dietetic Association, 92*(8), 996-1005.

Angell, N. (1990). Prisoners of technology. The case of Nancy Cruzan. *New England Journal of Medicine, 322*(17), 1226-1228.

Gaspar, P. M. (1988). What determines how much patients drink? *Geriatric Nursing, 9*, 221-224.

The Hastings Center. (1987). *Guidelines on the termination of life-sustaining treatment*. Briarcliff Manor, NY.

The Hastings Center guidelines for foregoing treatment. (1988). *Clinical Ethics Report, 2*, 1-8.

Institute of Medical Ethics. (1991). Working Party on Ethics of Prolonging Life and Assisted Death. Withdrawal of life support from patients in a persistent vegetative state. *Lancet, 337*, 96-98.

Keohane, P., Brown, B., & Gremble, G. (1981). The peptide nitrogen source of elemental diets: Comparison of absorptive properties of five partial enzyme hydrolyzates of a whole protein. *Journal of Parenteral and Enteral Nutrition, 5*, 568.

Koshuta, M. A., Schmitz, P. J., & Lynn, J. (1991, June). Development of an institutional policy on artificial nutrition and hydration. *Kennedy Institute of Ethics Journal*, p. 133-140.

Lavizzo-Mourey, R., Johnson, J., & Stolley, P. (1988). Risk factors for dehydration among elderly nursing home residents. *Journal of the American Geriatric Society, 36*, 213-218.

Lowe, B., McLeod, G. A., & Saika, G. (1986). Patient attitude toward discussing life-sustaining treatment. *Archives of Internal Medicine, 146*, 1613-1615.

Lowe, B., Rouse, F., & Dornband, L. (1990). Family decision making on trial. Who decides for incompetent patients? *New England Journal of Medicine, 322*(17), 1228-1232.

Lin, E. M. (1991). Nutrition support: Making the difficult decisions. *Cancer Nursing, 14*(5), 261-269.

Luce, J. M. (1990). Ethical principles in critical care. *Journal of the American Medical Association, 263*(5), 696-700.

Mahowald, J. M., & Himmelstein, D. U. (1981). Hypernutremia: Relation to infection and mortality. *Journal of the American Geriatric Society, 29*, 177-180.

Nancy Beth Cruzan v. Director, Missouri Department of Health, No. 88-1503, Daily Appellate Report, June 27, 1990.

National Research Council. (1989). *Recommended dietary allowances*. Washington, DC: National Academy Press.

Oley Foundation. (1985, November) *Nutritional support and hydration for critically and terminally ill elderly*. Prepared for the Office of Technology Assessment, United States Congress, Washington, DC

President's Commission for the Study of Ethical Problems in Medicine and Behavioral Research. (1981). *Defining death*. Washington, DC: U.S. Government Printing Office.

President's Commission for the Study of Ethical Problems in Medicine and Behavioral Research. (1983). *Deciding to forego life-sustaining treatment*. Washington, DC: U.S. Government Printing Office.

Raffin, T. A. (1991). Withholding and withdrawing life support. *Hospital Practice*, *26*, 133-155.

Rombeau, J., & Caldwell, M. (1984). *Clinical nutrition Volume 2: Parenteral nutrition*. Philadelphia, PA: W.B. Saunders Co.

Rombeau, J., & Caldwell, M. (1990). *Clinical nutrition: Enteral and tube feeding* (2nd ed.). Philadelphia, PA: W.B. Saunders Co.

Ruark, J. E., & Raffin, T. A. (1988). Initiating and withdrawing life support. Principles and practice in adult medicine. *New England Journal of Medicine*, *318*(1), 25-30.

Silk, D. B., Fairclough, P. D., & Clark, M. L. (1980). Use of a peptide rather than free amino acid nitrogen source in chemically defined "elemental diets." *Journal of Parenteral and Enteral Nutrition*, *4*, 548-553.

Singer, P. A., & Siegler, M. (1991). Elective use of life-sustaining treatment in internal medicine. *Archives of Internal Medicine*, *36*, 57-79.

Smedira, N. G., Evans, B. H., Grais, L. S., Cohen, N. H., Lowe, B., Cooke, M., Schechter, W. P., Fink, C., Epstein-Jaffe, E., May, C., & Luce, J. M. (1990). Withholding and withdrawal of life support from the critically ill. *New England Journal of Medicine*, *322*(5), 309-315.

Sprung, C. L. (1990). Changing attitudes and practices in foregoing life-sustaining treatments. *Journal of the American Medical Association*, *263*(16), 2211-2215.

Supreme Court Opinions (1991). Nancy Beth Cruzan, Petitioners v. Director, Missouri Department of Health et al. Full text of opinions in: *United States Law Week*, *58*, 4916-4941.

Stanley, J. M. (1989). The Appleton Consensus: Suggested international guidelines for decisions to forego medical treatment. *Journal of Medical Ethics*, *15*, 129-136.

Uhlmann, R. F., & Pearlman, R. A. (1991). Perceived quality of life and preferences for life-sustaining treatment in older adults. *Archives of Internal Medicine*, *151*, 495-497.

Young, E. A., Perkins, H. S., & McCamish, M. A. (1992). Ethical dimensions and clinical decisions for parenteral nutrition: In dying as in living. In J. L. Rombeau, & M. D. Caldwell (Eds.), *Clinical nutrition: Parenteral nutrition* (2nd ed.). Orlando, FL: W. B. Saunders.

Legal Decisions Affecting the Limitation of Nutritional Support

Eugene V. Boisaubin

SUMMARY. The withholding of nutritional support from patients is one of the most controversial issues in modern medical ethics and law. Withholding support from a consenting, terminally ill patient is the simplest case situation to defend, but patients in a persistent vegetative state or irreversible, chronic illness, require more careful deliberation. Regarding this issue, five primary principles have been utilized in legal decision making. These include: futility, autonomy, integrity of health professionals, states interests, balancing benefits versus harm and quality of life. The two landmark legal cases which have set the tone for most other court decisions are Paul Brophy and Nancy Beth Cruzan. Both cases clarified the right of competent adults to refuse nutritional support, even if life-saving. In the Cruzan case, however, states were given the authority to request clear and convincing evidence for the previous wishes of the incompetent patient. In summary, competent patients entering a hospice program should make informed decisions about their desires for feeding, as they do with other treatment decisions. Optimally, those wishes should be codified into an advance directive and a proxy decision maker named. If a patient is not competent, and without previously expressed wishes, immediate family members are usually consulted for what they believe are the patient's best interests. Last, although

---

Eugene V. Boisaubin, MD, is Associate Professor, Department of Internal Medicine, Medical Branch at Galveston, TX.

Address correspondence to: Eugene V. Boisaubin, MD, Department of Medicine, Rm. 4.156, University of Texas Medical Branch at Galveston, Galveston, TX 77555-0572.

[Haworth co-indexing entry note]: "Legal Decisions Affecting the Limitation of Nutritional Support." Boisaubin, Eugene V. Co-published simultaneously in *The Hospice Journal* (The Haworth Press, Inc.) Vol. 9, Nos. 2/3, 1993, pp. 131-147: and: *Nutrition and Hydration in Hospice Care: Needs, Strategies, Ethics* (eds: Gallagher-Allred, Charlette, and Madalon O'Rawe Amenta) The Haworth Press, Inc., 1993, pp. 131-147. Multiple copies of this article/chapter may be purchased from The Haworth Document Delivery Center [1-800-3-HAWORTH; 9:00 a.m. - 5:00 p.m. (EST)].

© 1993 by The Haworth Press, Inc. All rights reserved. *131*

limitations of care for terminally ill children fall under the same general guidelines as for adults, the "Baby Doe Rules" are a complicating factor.

INTRODUCTION

The potential withholding of food and fluids from patients has become one of the most controversial and intensely debated issues in modern biomedical ethics and law (Ahronheim & Gasner, 1990; Boisaubin, 1984; Dresser & Boisaubin, 1985; Lynn & Childress, 1983; Nelson, 1987; Siegler & Weisbard, 1985). The origins of this, and other medical and legal dilemmas that have surfaced in the past twenty years, are primarily in the scientific and technological advances that permit essential life processes to be maintained during critical and even in chronic illnesses. Respirator support, kidney dialysis, and nutritional support, such as enteral nutrition and total parenteral nutrition (TPN), share the common value of providing substantial benefit for patients with correctable illnesses. But they also share the common problem of allowing existence at some level to be maintained, almost indefinitely, even though the benefit of that existential state to the individual patient may be minimal or nonexistent.

For the clinician, a case involving a truly terminal patient–the prognosis of terminality can be made with relative certainty and death will result in the foreseeable future regardless of treatment–is probably the easiest situation in which to justify limitations of technologic support such as artificial feeding and hydration.

The term foreseeable, often poorly defined even by the courts, usually implies a period of hours, days or weeks, not months or years. The most obvious moral, medical, and legal justification for this limitation would be the concept of futility. If death is inevitable and treatment will have no impact, then aggressive forms of therapy, among them artificial feeding, may not be required since they can provide no true benefit (Younger, 1988). On the other hand, if a dying patient is still alert and expresses an interest in being fed, then food and hydration should be provided as desired, optimally by the simplest method–orally.

The two most difficult clinical situations involving feeding, those that have also been the focus of the most intense legal controversy, include patients who are in a persistent vegetative state, and patients who have chronic debilitating conditions, such as Alzheimer's disease. In the former, although the brainstem is intact and cardiopulmonary function is maintained, the cerebral cortex is not functioning and awareness is not present (Councils on Scientific Affairs and Ethical and Judicial Affairs, 1990). In the latter, there may be some awareness, but the quality of life is poor. In both situations, aggressive medical treatment including artificial feeding may sustain life for months or even years.

In another article in this issue, Dr. Mark McCamish addresses some of the ethical and practical issues surrounding decisions to provide enteral and parenteral nutritional support to terminally ill patients (Councils on Scientific Affairs and Ethical and Judicial Affairs, 1990). In the remainder of this paper, I will first outline some of the general legal principles that have been the foundation for decisions concerning limitation of feeding and provide historical context. I will then describe in detail two of the most important cases in the past decade that have had the greatest impact on our current legal system concerning limitation of medical treatment in general, and specifically, issues of nutritional support. The first case is that of Paul Brophy of Massachusetts and the second is that of Nancy Beth Cruzan of Missouri. The implications of these court decisions will then be brought together to create summary recommendations and guidelines to assist health care workers, and specifically hospice personnel, who deal with end-of-life nutrition and hydration issues.

GENERAL LEGAL PRINCIPLES

Futility

Although many of the controversies discussed above have originated in recent advances in science and technology, the ethical and legal principles they invoke are long standing (see Table I). The first and fundamental principle of futility has already been addressed in this volume (McCamish & Crocker). Courts have generally agreed

TABLE I

**Ethical and Legal Principles Used in
Court Deliberations About
Limitation of Nutritional Support**

- Futility
- Autonomy
- Integrity of Health
  Professionals
- State's Interest
- Balancing Benefit
  versus Harm
- Quality Of life

that health professionals are under no obligation to provide treatment that is of no benefit, particularly if the patient is terminally ill (Younger, 1988).

Autonomy

The second and perhaps more important principle is the concept of autonomy or self determination, which is deeply rooted in our culture. In general, this is the moral right to choose and follow one's own plan of life and action (Beauchamp & Childress, 1989). Legally, these preferences are significant because the American legal system recognizes that individuals have a fundamental right to control their own bodies, and the right to be protected from unwanted interventions. An important judicial opinion, that of *Natanson v. Kline* (1960) maintains:

> Anglo American law starts with the premise of thoroughgoing self-determination. It follows that each man is considered to be master of his own body, and he may, if he be of sound mind, prohibit the performance of life saving surgery or other medical treatment. (Jonsen, Siegler, & Winslade, 1992, p. 39)

For example, a competent, adult terminally ill patient has the right to refuse placement of an intravenous catheter for chemotherapy if he or she feels that it is not in his or her best interest.

When the patient is no longer competent and has failed to complete a written advance directive, the issue of what she or he would want becomes more complex. This critical void was the center of considerable controversy in the Cruzan decision.

Integrity of Health Care Workers

A third legal principle is the integrity of the health care workers involved in the treatment process. Although the competent adult patient has great power in deciding whether to accept or refuse medical treatment, it is both inappropriate and unethical to force health care providers to violate their own professional and ethical standards. For example, a health care provider may object to the withholding of dialysis or nutritional support that he or she believes is essential to maintain existing life and which when stopped, will directly result in death. Just as an obstetrician or a nurse with strong moral convictions against abortion should not be required to participate in such a procedure, health professionals have the option to refuse to participate in treatment decisions they believe will end life or increase suffering. An institution such as a religiously sponsored hospital, might also codify this principle into hospital policy by categorically refusing to terminate nutritional support in any patient, unless there is clear medical indication.

State's Interest

A fourth legal principle would be the issue of the state's interest in maintaining individual life. This concept, very old in English common law, argues that the king as the earthly surrogate of God, has the right to prohibit suicide or the taking of life because this constitutes an "offense to God" and/or deprives the king of a taxable, intact citizen (De Prerogativa Regis, 1324). Although some contend that the government still tries to usurp powers belonging only to God, this argument is infrequently used. On the other hand, it has become an issue in some right-to-die cases, such as Cruzan, since the State of Missouri argued that it had a vested or compelling interest in maintaining the life of each of its citizens.

Benefit versus Burden

Another legal principle that has been drawn into the feeding debate is the balancing of benefit versus harm. For example, would the implementation of TPN be of overall benefit to a terminally ill patient when the risks–line placement, sepsis, metabolic complications–are weighed against the potential benefit of improved nutritional status and perhaps prolongation of life?

Quality of Life

Last, the issue of quality of life has periodically been addressed by the courts. This concept is fraught with problems because of the subjectivity and human variability involved in its determination. For example, many people while healthy, when questioned, would reject the prospect of continued life with a profound disability such as quadriplegia. On the other hand, the majority living with this condition desire to go on living rather than request death.

HISTORICAL CONTEXT

The history of legal cases involving withdrawal of medical care is a short one, spanning only twenty years. The first important case to achieve both widespread public awareness and legal precedent, that of Karen Ann Quinlan, was decided in 1976 (*In re* Quinlan, 1976). Miss Quinlan lapsed into a persistent vegetative state after a drug overdose and subsequently her family requested, and permission was granted, to discontinue her respirator support. Interestingly, withdrawal of nutritional support by enteral feeding was not an issue in the decision since the family did not request it. With nutritional support, Miss Quinlan lived for more than ten additional years until her death in 1981. Her tragic life provided not only a legal landmark, but also evidence of how long life can be continued when excellent medical care, including nutritional support is maintained.

PAUL BROPHY

The Brophy Case

Paul E. Brophy, Sr., a former fire fighter and an emergency medical technician had unsuccessfully undergone surgery in April of 1983 for a ruptured basilar artery aneurysm and never regained consciousness (Steinbrook & Lo, 1988). In a persistent vegetative state in June of that year, he was transferred to a convalescent hospital. After further medical complications his physicians and his wife, who was also his legal guardian, agreed that he not be resuscitated in the event of a cardiac arrest. In December Mrs. Brophy consented to the placement of a gastrostomy feeding tube.

On a number of occasions prior to his terminal illness Mr. Brophy had repeatedly told family members to "pull the plug" if he should ever end up in a coma. At another time he became angry after having received a commendation for pulling a man from a burning truck, only to learn that the man had suffered greatly before dying several months later. Although Mr. Brophy had made repeated general statements about not wanting to be kept alive in a comatose condition, he never specifically mentioned artificial feeding.

Mr. Brophy's condition remained unchanged through 1984, at which time Mrs. Brophy felt that his active life was over and in view of his previously expressed wishes, began to question the provision of artificial feeding. After consultation with clergy, an ethicist, and a lawyer, she requested that the feeding be stopped. The couple's children and other family members were supportive of the decision, but Mr. Brophy's personal physician and the hospital administration were opposed.

In February of 1985, Mrs. Brophy asked a probate court to allow her husband's tube feeding to be discontinued and in December, the judge ruled against her. The judge, however, did state that Mr. Brophy would rather be dead than have his life prolonged in a persistent vegetative state. Mrs. Brophy appealed, and in September of 1986, the Massachusetts Supreme Judicial Court held in a four to three decision that Paul Brophy's feeding tube could be removed. The United States Supreme Court declined to review the decision.

The following month, Mr. Brophy was transferred to a nearby

hospital, under the care of a neurologist who had testified that Brophy was in a persistent vegetative state. Plans for supportive care were coordinated with Mrs. Brophy. On October 23, 1986, eight days after the tube feeding was discontinued, Paul Brophy died of pneumonia with his wife and children at the bedside.

The Brophy Decision

The Massachusetts Supreme Judicial Court ruled that Brophy's tube feeding could be discontinued as he would have wished (*Brophy v. New England*, 1986). The decision was based on common law and the presumed constitutional right of patients to refuse medical treatment, regardless of the views of others. It also rejected the argument that artificial feeding should be continued because it represented ordinary rather than extraordinary care. In addition, the court rejected a distinction between withholding and withdrawing treatments, including artificial feeding. They argued that if stopping treatment is viewed as more difficult than not starting it, this distinction could discourage attempts to begin needed treatment and lead to premature decisions to allow patients to die. The court also said that Brophy's right to refuse medical treatments, including artificial feeding, outweighed both state interests that might favor continuing treatment and the ethical integrity of the medical profession. Concerning the preservation of life, the court argued that the state had no duty to preserve life when the patient felt that the means of doing so demeaned his humanity. Only Paul Brophy could make decisions about the quality of his life and physicians or third parties including the court, did not have that power. Although he was not terminally ill, the court determined that he still had the right to refuse life-sustaining treatments including artificial feeding. The court also felt that this decision would not subject Brophy to a painful death by starvation. Instead, his choice would allow the underlying disease to take its natural course. Last, the majority decision concluded that the ethical integrity of the medical profession would not be violated as long as health care providers were not compelled to discontinue feeding against their will. The court acknowledged, however, that the hospital could not be forced to withhold artificial feeding if such action ran contrary to their views or patient care policies. Mrs. Brophy, therefore, was assisted in arranging transfer to another institution where her wishes could be carried out.

Three judges dissented. Their arguments included that state interest in the preservation of life had not been given appropriate weight; that the decision sanctioned the individual's right to commit suicide; and that providing food and fluids was not medical treatment, but a more basic human need that should always be met.

The Brophy Case: Summary

In summary, the Brophy case was a significant decision in a number of ways. The state court majority reaffirmed the common law rights of individuals and assumed the constitutional right of refusal of medical treatments including artificial feeding. Factors making this decision even more remarkable were that the patient was not terminally ill, he was not competent, and he had not completed a written advance directive. This right of refusal was given precedence over other competing claims, including the state's interest in preserving life and the objections of some of the health care providers involved in the case. Mr. Brophy's previous statements were given considerable weight as was the input of his family. The case was also noteworthy in the reliance of the justices upon the authority of a number of medical professional groups, such as the American Medical Association, The American Academy of Neurology, and the Massachusetts Medical Society, all of which deemed removal of artificial feeding from such patients as ethical (Ahronheim & Gasner, 1990).

NANCY BETH CRUZAN

The Cruzan case has become the single most important decision in American law addressing the general issue of withdrawal of medical care, and specifically the issue of termination of nutritional support. It was the only case of this type to reach the United States Supreme Court (*Cruzan v. Director*, 1990). The details of this involved case have been exhaustively discussed elsewhere (Lo & Steinbrook, 1991) and only a brief summary will be provided here.

The Cruzan Case

Nancy Cruzan was a thirty-three year old woman who was severely injured in an automobile accident in rural Missouri in January of 1983. She was resuscitated and respiration and heartbeat, but not consciousness, were restored. Maintained by food and water through a gastrostomy tube, she remained in a persistent vegetative state. After several years, all of her physicians and consultants agreed that she would not recover.

In 1987, Miss Cruzan's parents requested that their daughter's feeding tube be removed, in part on the basis of her statement that she would not want to continue to live if she could not be "at least half normal." A trial judge agreed with her parents' request, but the Missouri Supreme Court overturned the decision by pronouncing that Miss Cruzan's right to refuse treatment was hers alone and no one could exercise it for her. The court argued that clear and convincing evidence was necessary that she would have rejected such treatment since the consequence of stopping nutrition and hydration was death, and because the state had legitimate interests in preserving life.

The Cruzan Decision

Miss Cruzan's parents appealed the decision to the United States Supreme Court where it was argued in 1989 and decided five to four, in June of 1990. The majority opinion held that competent patients have a "constitutionally protected liberty interest in refusing unwanted medical treatment" under the due process clause in the fourteenth amendment to the Constitution. The Court stated, however, that incompetent patients did not have the same right because they cannot directly exercise it. Therefore, states are permitted to establish more stringent procedural safeguards governing medical decisions for incompetent patients than are in effect for competent patients.

The majority opinion declared that the individual's right to refuse treatment must be balanced against relevant state interests, including "the protection and preservation of human life." It also ruled that the Constitution allows states to establish procedures to prevent abuses, to exclude quality of life as a consideration of treatment decisions, and to err on the side of continuing life-sustaining treatment. In essence, states may require life sustaining treatment when there is no clear and convincing evidence that the incompetent patient would have refused it. The Court, however, did agree that Cruzan's condition would not improve and that the available evidence about her preferences suggested that she would not want further tube feedings.

In dissent, three justices argued that being free of unwanted medical treatment is a fundamental constitutional right and it extends to incompetent as well as competent patients, and that this right includes refusal of artificial nutrition and fluid. Two of the justices argued that the fundamental right to refuse treatment could not be overridden by the more general issue of "state's interests."

After the Supreme Court ruling, the Cruzans petitioned the trial court of Missouri to rehear their request to discontinue tube feeding, arguing that new witnesses had come forward who had had specific discussions with Nancy before her accident about her wishes for life sustaining treatment. In November of 1990 a new hearing was held in which two women who had worked with Nancy in 1978 stated that in their conversations with her she had made specific statements about not wanting to be kept alive as a "vegetable."

In December, a state judge authorized Cruzan's parents to "cause the removal" of artificial feedings, arguing that Cruzan's intent, "if medically able, would be to terminate her nutrition and hydration." The Attorney General of Missouri asked that the state be withdrawn from the court decision at this time because he felt that the remaining parties would follow the legal "clear and convincing" evidence guidelines enunciated by the U.S. Supreme Court. The tube feedings were stopped almost immediately and Miss Cruzan died 12 days later.

The Cruzan Case: Summary

In summary, the U.S. Supreme Court decision can be interpreted in a variety of ways. First and perhaps most important, the Court majority reaffirmed that the U.S. Constitution protects refusal of life sustaining treatment by competent patients. Individual states, however, may impose procedural safeguards for incompetent patients to insure that their specific wishes, if they can be determined, will be carried out.

However, continuation of tube feeding for Miss Cruzan, who remained in a persistent vegetative state, was supported. This continuation was in opposition to the patient's wishes as well as her family's. This part of the decision is in obvious contrast with the Brophy decision, which respected previous wishes by the patient to justify termination of treatment. The Cruzan ruling directly rejected the traditional practice of respecting family decision making for incompetent patients.

The Supreme Court also left much of the future decision making about limiting treatment to the individual states. The Cruzan decision applies to Missouri only. The ruling elaborates that other states may adopt similar guidelines, but there is no requirement to do so. Unfortunately, state law and precedent vary tremendously. Some states allow families to refuse treatment on behalf of incompetent terminally ill patients. Many states, however, have no policies or laws regarding family decision making for incompetent patients. Health care providers will always need to clarify the nature of existing, relevant state law (Thomasma, 1991).

CONCLUSIONS AND GUIDELINES FOR DEALING WITH END OF LIFE ISSUES

This summary of general legal principles and two important recent cases provides some general guidelines for health care practitioners dealing with end-of-life issues. Although variations in court decisions exist, a number of consistent legal trends can be noted. Perhaps most important and consistent is the court's respect for the rights of competent, adult individuals to reject medical care, even when it is life sustaining. This acceptance of patients' wishes is perhaps strongest when terminal conditions are clearly present, the proposed treatment can be defined as futile, and death can be foreseen. Fortunately for the hospice worker, these kinds of circumstances should characterize the great majority of patients cared for in a hospice setting.

Ideally, the patient should be alert and have the capacity to decide his or her treatment goals in a rational fashion with professional input. These discussions are best undertaken at the earliest time possible in the course of a terminal illness when the patient is better able to reflect on the implications of the decision.

After discussion and decision making have taken place, it is optimal to codify the decisions into a written document, such as an advance directive or living will, now accepted in almost all of the fifty states (Annas, 1990; Singer & Siegler, 1992). The relevant state document should be carefully inspected to see if issues of termination of feeding are specifically addressed. The competent patient can then sign the advance directive, indicating a willingness to limit, in general, non-beneficial end-of-life treatments. If they are not cited in the general document, individual treatments, such as respirator support, dialysis, or nutritional support, might be specifically listed and added for greater clarification.

Family awareness, and perhaps even input into an advance directive is advisable, if it is desired by the patient. Although the competent adult has the right to make such a decision on his or her own, it is optimal that the family be aware of the written directive so that lack of knowledge and disagreement do not restrict its later use. The appropriate witnesses, as indicated by state law, should be utilized and several copies of the document should be made. Copies should be retained by the patient, designated family members, the primary treating physician, and the treating institution as part of the medical record.

The Patient Self Determination Act

The use of advance directives has been facilitated by the Patient Self Determination Act, effective December 1, 1991, requiring health care institutions to question and inform patients about these provisions. The law specifically requires that patients entering a medical institution receiving federal funds for medical services be questioned about whether they have an advance directive already prepared (Omnibus Bill, 1990). If so, this information must be documented in the patient's chart. The law also requires the medical institution to inform the patient of its own policies and relevant state law concerning the existence and availability of these instruments. The law is intended to encourage education and awareness about this issue and does not require a patient to complete an advance directive.

Proxy Option

Another option, sometimes part of the advance directive, is to have the competent patient name a proxy to assist in medical decision making if and when he or she becomes incompetent. Many regard this as the preferred approach since even a well informed person cannot begin to anticipate all of the end-of-life issues that may arise as competency wanes. The health care professional and/or institution can then turn to the designated adult proxy for input. Some states have codified this approach and have established a medical power of attorney form which may be used in addition to or in conjunction with a traditional advance directive (Emanuel & Emanuel, 1992).

The Optimal Process

In summary, the optimal way for a patient to make end-of-life decisions about medical treatments, including continuation of feeding, is to make a clear informed decision when competent, discuss this with family and health providers, and then codify these wishes into a formal advance directive, perhaps with the addition of a designated proxy decision maker.

Incompetent Patients Without Advance Directives

For the incompetent patient, who has not completed an advance directive, the legal issues and options are less clear. A number of states have laws that allow for an involved family to make end-of-life decisions, based on what they believe to be the patient's beliefs or best interests (Lo & Steinbrook, 1991). Although immediate family input is usually respected in almost all health care settings, the Cruzan decision stated that in certain situations, states might be able to override family input if clear and convincing evidence of patient desires could not be provided. The individual health practitioner or institution needs to refer to current state law or policy.

Patients in Vegetative States

For patients who are not obviously terminally ill, or who may be in a vegetative state, the guidelines are even less clear. Again, for the patient who has previously documented his or her wishes in an advance directive, these guidelines should be adequate. There are, however, exceptions. Missouri law does not allow patients to refuse "any procedure to provide nutrition or hydration" through a living will. The constitutionality of this portion of the law, however, is questionable. In the Cruzan case, although the Court did not specifically rule on the issue, five U.S. Supreme Court Justices interpreted the Constitution as protecting refusal of artificial feeding.

Institutional Policy

In general, it would seem to be advisable that if health care institutions have strong beliefs about the difficult issues that surround limitations of artificial feeding, they should develop a formal, written policy. This would not only benefit future patients and aid institutional decision making, but the resulting necessary active dialogue among health professionals would facilitate education and understanding of all involved.

TERMINALLY ILL CHILDREN

Lastly, children with irreversible illnesses constitute a unique set of problems. In general, proposals to limit or withdraw medical treatment with children follow the same professional and ethical guidelines as with adults, the obvious exception being that the child is usually viewed as not having the capacity to participate in the decision. Some children, notably adolescents, may demonstrate sufficient insight and comprehension that a court will hear and even accept their viewpoint.

"Baby Doe Rules"

Limitation of care for pediatric patients is also delineated in the 1985 Congressional Amendment entitled "The Child Abuse Pre-

vention and Treatment and Adoption Reform Act," commonly
known as the "Baby Doe Rules." Observance of these standards is
monitored by State Child Protective Agencies. The regulations read
that treatment is not required, "when the provision of such treatment would merely prolong dying, not be effective in ameliorating
or correcting all of the infant's life conditions, or otherwise be futile
in terms of the survival of the infant" (Public Law, 1984). The
"Baby Doe Rules," however, require artificial feeding to be continued, even in terminal conditions. In these most difficult cases,
institutional legal counsel is most advisable if any limitation in
nutritional support for children is contemplated.

REFERENCES

Ahronheim, J., & Gasner, M. (1990). The sloganism of starvation. *Lancet, 335*,
278-279.
Annas, G. J. (1990). Nancy Cruzan and the right to die. *New England Journal of
Medicine, 323*(10), 78-80.
Beauchamp, T. L., & Childress, J. F. (1989). *Principles of biomedical ethics*. New
York: Oxford University Press.
Boisaubin, E. (1984). Ethical issues in the nutritional support of the terminal
patient. *Journal of the American Dietetic Association, 84*(5), 529-31.
Brophy v. New England Sinai Hospital, Inc., 497 N.E.2d. 626 (Mass. 1986).
Councils on Scientific Affairs and Ethical and Judicial Affairs. (1990). Persistent
vegetative state and the decision to withdraw or withhold life support. *Journal
of the American Medical Association, 263*(3), 426-30.
Cruzan v. Director, Missouri Department of Health, 110 S. Ct 2841 (1990).
De Prerogativa Regis. (1324).
Dresser, R., & Boisaubin, E. (1985). Ethics, law and nutritional support. *Archives
of Internal Medicine, 145*, 122-124.
Emanuel, E. J., & Emanuel, L. L. (1992). Proxy decision making for incompetent
patients–an ethical and empirical analysis. *Journal of the American Medical
Association, 67*(15), 2067-2071.
In re Quinlan, 355 A 2d 647 (N.J. 1976).
Jonsen, A. R., Siegler, M., & Winslade, W. J. (1992). *Clinical ethics* (3rd ed.).
New York: McGraw-Hill.
Lo, B., & Steinbrook, R. (1991). Beyond the Cruzan case–the U.S. Supreme Court
and medical practice. *Annals of Internal Medicine, 114*, 895-901.
Lynn, J., & Childress, J. F. (1983). Must patients always be given food and water?
Hastings Center Report, 13(5), 17-21.
McCamish, M. A., & Crocker, N. J. (1993). Enteral and parenteral nutrition
support of terminally ill patients: Practical and ethical perspective. *The Hos-
pice Journal, 9*(2,3).

Nelson, L. J. (1987). Foregoing nutrition and hydration. *Clinical Ethics Report*, *1*(1), 1-7.

(Omnibus Bill) Omnibus Budget Reconciliation Act 1990. Title 4, Section 4206. *Congressional Record*, October 26, 12638, 1990.

Public Law, 98-457, October 9, 1984.

Siegler, M., & Weisbard, A. (1985). Against the emerging stream: Should fluid and nutritional support be discontinued? *Archives of Internal Medicine*, *145*, 129-131.

Singer, P. A., & Siegler, M. (1992). Advancing the cause of advance directives. *Archives of Internal Medicine*, *152*, 22-24.

Steinbrook, R., & Lo, B. (1988). Artificial feeding–solid ground, not a slippery slope. *New England Journal of Medicine*, *318*, 286-290.

Thomasma, D. C. (1991). The Cruzan decision and medical practice. *Archives of Internal Medicine*, *151*, 853-854.

Younger, S. J. (1988). Who defines futility? *Journal of the American Medical Association*, *260*, 2094-2095.

Index

Abandonment fears, 37
Acceptance and food quality, 97
Acquired immune deficiency
    syndrome *See* AIDS
Adult care
    assessment form for, 42-45
    enteral/parenteral nutrition and, 40
    ethical issues in, 47,51-53
    guidelines for, 40-41,46-47
    hospice dietitian in, 38-39
Advance directives, 47
    absence of, 140-141,144
Agitated patients, 49
Aguilera, D. C., 6,7
Ahronheim, J., 132,139
AIDS, 77,79,110
    anorexia in, 75
    foodservice issues, 102-103
Allen, K. S., 2
Allen-Masterson, S., 13,15
Alternative therapies, 62
Alzheimer's disease, 133
AMA Councils on Scientific Affairs
    and Ethical and Judicial
    Affairs, 133
Ambiguity, 11-12
Amenta, C., 16
Amenta, M. O., 19,86
American Academy of Neurology,
    139
American Dietetic Association
    (ADA), 39,51,52,
    105,123-125
American Heart Association, 115
American Medical Association
    (AMA), 51,133,139
American Nurses Association
    (ANA), 51

American Society of Parenteral and
    Enteral Nutrition ASPEN),
    119-120
Amyotrophic lateral sclerosis (ALS),
    109
Analgesia
    and appetite, 80-81
    dehydration as, 4-5,28
    narcotic and fiber requirements, 116
    side effects of narcotic, 81
Andrews, M. R., 26
Angell, N., 108
Annas, G. J., 143
Anorexia, 13-14,41
    in cancer, 18-19,22-23
    in children, 64
    and depression, 81
    etiology of, 74-75
    and gastric motility, 81
    medical treatment, 77-80
    physical effects of, 73-74
    symptom management and, 80-82
Antiemetics, 21
Armbruster, G., 94
Artificial nutrition *See* Hydration
    therapy; Nutrition
    intervention; Parenteral
    nutrition
Ascites, 28
Ashwal, S., 70
ASPEN guidelines, 119-120
Assessment
    of adults, 41,42-45
    of cancer patient and family, 18-19
    of children, 57,58
    of foodservice performance, 98
    screening, 19,20
Autonomy, 134-135

© 1993 by The Haworth Press, Inc. All rights reserved. *149*